Scholarly Writing

Scholarly Writing

Techniques to Transcend Nurses' Notes

PEARMAN D. PARKER, PhD, MPH, RN, PMH-BC

ELIZABETH RILEY, DNP, APRN, CPNP-AC, PED-BC, RNC-NIC, CNE, ANEF

University of Arkansas for Medical Sciences

cognella®
SAN DIEGO

Bassim Hamadeh, CEO and Publisher
Amanda Martin, Publisher
Amy Smith, Senior Project Editor
Abbey Hastings, Production Editor
Emely Villavicencio, Senior Graphic Designer
Kylie Bartolome, Licensing Coordinator
Kim Scott/Bumpy Design, Interior Designer
Natalie Piccotti, Director of Marketing
Kassie Graves, Senior Vice President, Editorial
Jamie Giganti, Director of Academic Publishing

cognella® ACADEMIC PUBLISHING
320 South Cedros Ave., Ste. 400, Solana Beach, CA 92075

Brief Contents

Detailed Contents

Preface

Nurses are enrolling in graduate nursing programs at an exponential rate. The increasing enrollment for PhD, DNP, and MSN programs reflects students' desires to increase their clinical and scientific knowledge with the goal of leading the field of nursing. However, newly enrolled students face a major obstacle—scholarly writing. Graduate nursing students are expected to write well in graduate school, but most associate and baccalaureate programs place little emphasis on scholarly writing. Instead, the focii are on nursing skills and critical thinking application. Additionally, graduate nursing students often have a clinical background where the only writing emphasis is on documentation. As a result, graduate nursing students are often underprepared to meet the demands of scholarly writing in graduate school.

The mission of our writing workbook is to prepare graduate nursing students with basic knowledge and skills to embark on the scholarly writing process with joy and optimism. We use adult learning theory principles to guide graduate nursing students through scholarly writing principles and concepts. We also draw on our own unique blend of personal and clinical experiences to teach foundational scholarly writing skills.

Our workbook is designed to guide students through the scholarly writing process by focusing on topics such as organization, paraphrasing, grammar, and peer review. We include many interactive features in our book through the strategic use of writing prompts and journaling using self-reflection. We also incorporate real-life advice from other researchers, nurses, and educators to offer graduate nursing students a realistic perspective on the challenges and rewards of scholarly writing.

Collectively, we would like to acknowledge and thank the support of our own College of Nursing at the University of Arkansas for Medical Sciences. We received invaluable support of our dean and professor, Dr. Patricia Cowan, and our program director for Accreditation and College Affairs who is also our in-house film scholar and writing guru, Dr. Chris Dumas. Both believed in our endeavor and supported our time to devote to this project.

Individually, we would like to express the following:

Thank you to my father and first editor, Dr. James V. Parker, Jr., who showed me how to see beauty in writing and find persistence in editing. Also thank you to my mother, Suzanne deTreville, who poured endless encouragement over me. Lastly, I'd like to dedicate this book to all my past, current, and future nursing students. I am so honored to be part of your graduate school experiences.

Pearman D. Parker, PhD, MPH, RN, PMH-BC

I would like to thank all of my mentors and colleagues throughout my career who have shaped me into the writer that I am today. Additionally, to my family, thank you for your continuous encouragement and support in making this project possible.

Elizabeth Riley, DNP, APRN, CPNP-AC,
PED-BC, RNC-NIC, CNE, ANEF

Reviewers

Toby J. Brooks
Texas Tech University Health Sciences Center

Denise C. De La Rosa, DNP, APRN, FNP-C
Texas Wesleyan University

Mark C. Hand, PhD, RN, CNE
East Carolina University College of Nursing, Greenville, North Carolina

Pamela Love, PhD, MSN, BSN, CNE

Jeanette A. McNeill, DrPH, MSN, CNE, ANEF
Professor Emeritus, University of Northern Colorado

Veronica Quattrini, DNP, MS, FNP-BC
Senior Director for the Doctor of Nursing Practice Program, University of Maryland, Baltimore, School of Nursing

Robin Redmon Wright, PhD
Pennsylvania State University, Harrisburg

CHAPTER 1

Taking a Holistic Approach

Acknowledging Attitudes Toward Scholarly Writing by Using a Self-Inventory

Pearman D. Parker and Elizabeth Riley

The demands of graduate school can be exhausting. The daily stress of balancing assignments, managing time, and maintaining personal obligations can negatively impact academic performance (Llego et al., 2018). As many as 90.6% of graduate students report experiencing at least one specific stressor during their course of study (Rocha Cesar et al., 2018). Additionally, graduate nursing students face another challenge unique to their field—working at the bedside while still a student. According to a report from the Georgetown University's Center on Education and the Workforce, more than 76% of graduate students work at least 30 hours per week (Carnevale et al., 2015). Graduate nursing students are no exception and often continue working at the bedside while enrolled in their program of study. While the data show conflicting evidence of positive and negative effects of employment on academic performance (Dundes & Marx, 2006; Pike et al., 2008), stress remains a constant obstacle to achieving academic success (Fonseca et al., 2019). One of the most challenging stressors affecting graduate nursing students is the process of perfecting academic, or scholarly, writing.

Scholarly writing equates to clear, concise, and compelling communication in which writers demonstrate critical thought (Edmunds & Waldrop, 2018). General rules for scholarly writing include using active voice, incorporating peer-reviewed references, and avoiding poor grammar. Further description of scholarly writing elements is included in Chapter 3. While the definitions of scholarly writing may appear straightforward, graduate nursing students often struggle to apply the rules and experience significant amounts of stress in the process (Micsinszki & Yeung, 2021). As a result, graduate students can experience a range in severity of anxiety and fear when embarking on a writing project (Wynne et al., 2014). Some students may procrastinate, whereas others may overcorrect and complete assignments far in advance. Most graduate nursing students overcome scholarly writing stress and complete their assignments, graduate, and continue to their professional careers. However, despite the appearance of mastery that accompanies the successful completion of writing assignments, the stress of the writing process can be a continuing obstacle unless the student takes action to improve their writing skills.

Depending on the institution's support system, graduate nursing students can choose tutoring, writing classes, or participation in small-group activities such as "Shut Up & Write" (Micsinszki & Yeung, 2021) to learn methods to improve their writing skills and reduce the stress associated with the process. Nursing faculty can also teach graduate students specific skills and rules required for acceptable scholarly writing. Regardless of the type of instruction, graduate nursing students face similar challenges and learn through a "filter" of feelings, motivations, and sense of self (Krashen, 1982). Krashen's (1982) classic use of this concept of a filter to teaching students a secondary language, and Alice Horning (1987) applies this definition to writing. Horning (1987) refers to students overcoming this mental filter as the "first main hurdle" to improving and refining writing skills. Feelings—most crucially, fear (of failure, of ridicule, etc.)—may be the most challenging (and the most easily amenable) hurdle for graduate nursing students to overcome in the effort to write in a scholarly mode.

The fear of scholarly writing is a broad description that encompasses any negative emotions surrounding the writing process. Emotions such as distress, dread, nervousness, and uneasiness can be troublesome to overcome. Additionally, the negative emotions can trigger anxiety and lead to physical symptoms such as stomach and chest pains (National Institute of Mental Health, 2018). The result may be total or intermittent paralysis and can lead some students to procrastinate (Haghbin et al., 2012). Further, graduate nursing students may not seek additional feedback from faculty on their assignments out of fear of criticism (Penn, 2016). Without the feedback from editors, peers, faculty, or other instructors, students are then robbed of the opportunity to revise and strengthen their work. This cycle can continue or repeat itself, and the fear of scholarly writing may grow with each written assignment. However, the fear and stress associated with scholarly writing—or with writing in general, as a mode of self-expression—often takes root long before the graduate course of study. Such events may occur in high school or as early as elementary school. Before a graduate nursing student can navigate and overcome the fear of writing, a thorough self-inventory of attitudes and beliefs toward writing is necessary. However, many students do not always take time to evaluate such underlying perspectives. Before students can begin to unpack the range of emotions and attitudes toward scholarly writing and apply helpful solutions (with a goal of becoming a stronger, more effective writer), students need to take a holistic, or widespread, approach to determine underlying attitudes.

First, a self-inventory is an ideal method to identify any preconceived notions, beliefs, and attitudes that may provide additional insight to graduate nursing students' current perspectives toward scholarly writing (Butcher, 2009). Often the self-inventory reveals more hidden perspectives that may originate from former coursework (as early as elementary school).

Second, acknowledging the influence of writing clinical nursing notes and reports can be equally informative. Identifying this mix of perspectives is critical to overcome and mitigate the fear of scholarly writing, which can ultimately lead to writing success.

Part 1: Identifying Writing Perspectives Using Self-Inventory Questions

Use the space provided to write in your answers, or brainstorm answers with peers—whatever works best for you.

- When you think of writing, what first comes to mind? *Write down your initial reactions and try to not think too hard. The goal is to freely express your associations without thought.*

  ____

  ____

  ____

  ____

- How many of these responses were associated with emotions? Did you come up with any words, such as *frustrating*? *Laborious*? Alternatively, what about *fun*? *Easy*?

  ____

  ____

  ____

  ____

You will need to be aware of, and monitor, the trends of your emotional response to a skill-based activity, such as writing.

- Next, how many of these responses are rooted in your *direct experience* with writing? In other words, what specific experiences from your past come to your memory when you think about the emotions surrounding writing?

  ____

  ____

  ____

  ____

- Write down a few key memories you associate with writing. *Try to list a variety of experiences, ranging from scary to exciting, from your childhood to college.*

  ____

  ____

  ____

  ____

- Out of the experiences listed, how many were rooted in relation to your experience with writing *as a nurse?*

  ____

  ____

  ____

  ____

Applying the Self-Inventory to Writing in Graduate School

This self-inventory of writing attitudes and experiences may be initially overwhelming. However, this process can reveal key perspectives, which lead to behaviors (procrastination, delay in seeking advice, etc.) that are critical to overcome in the writing process. Testing and implementing personalized strategies can be a useful method to overcome behaviors associated with the fear of scholarly writing (Silvia, 2019). Personalized strategies should be tailored to each student and to their unique writing perspectives and experiences identified from the self-inventory. Silvia (2019) offers useful strategies in his book *How to Write a Lot: A Practical Guide to Academic Writing*, which is recommended across graduate nursing programs. The suggestions are adapted and revised here:

For students who are overwhelmed with an assignment:

- Take three to five deep breaths to calm nervous system.
- Review assignment criteria gradually and make a plan for productivity.
  - Allow time for social events in your personal life.
  - Set aside time for feedback from external reviewers (e.g., faculty asking for a draft).
  - Be gentle with yourself if anything unexpected comes up.

For students who delay starting a writing assignment:

- Set a small goal (e.g., working on the title page).

- Start the writing process (making an outline, writing down ideas) by jotting notes down on actual paper (and not on a computer) to facilitate creativity.
- Make a date for your writing time (be intentional about setting a time and day in a special environment of your choosing).
- Reward yourself for sticking to your writing schedule.
- Give yourself grace if you miss a day or two of writing.

For students who thrive in social settings:

- Use structured weekly writing groups to meet with peers and write together.
- Choose a local coffee shop to be surrounded by others to reduce loneliness or add variety to your writing experience.
- Ask friends to help you be accountable for your own writing goals.

For students who are easily distracted:

- Turn off email alerts and silence phone notifications.
- Find quiet writing settings with reduced distractions (adequate room temperature, minimal opportunity for interacting with others, comfortable work settings).
- If possible, try to write during your own ideal productivity time (e.g., morning, afternoon, evening, etc.).
- Select a place to write that is positively associated with productivity. Make this your sacred writing space. Do not contaminate your writing space with other activities.

The key to using the writing self-inventory is to acknowledge the influence of the fear of scholarly writing on the process of writing. Graduate nursing students can then apply the strategies to mitigate and reduce their own writing fears.

Our hope is for students to use this workbook and gradually refine their attitudes and behaviors surrounding the writing process. We believe that when students are equipped to navigate their own fears and have the skills necessary for writing well, they are then able to reach their own levels of success in academic and professional settings.

Part 2: Identifying Writing Perspectives From Clinical Experiences and the Impact on Scholarly Writing

In addition to students' feelings, perceptions, and behaviors associated with scholarly writing, the clinical environment has an impact on scholarly writing beyond what students may realize. Quality scholarly writing and effective communication are interrelated concepts, and

Clinical Example 1

A friend once described the bubbles surrounding a patient's mouth as "frothy" in her nursing note. This sent our clinical instructor into a tizzy, and my friend accidentally sounded the alarm by insinuating that patient had frothy sputum. The reality was that the patient had some innocent mouth bubbles from some ill-fitting dentures. While my friend was trying to pick just one word ("frothy") to describe the bubbles, the context surrounding the word was not fitting (no pun intended). She restricted the use of extra descriptive words in her notes but struggled to elaborate in her academic papers due to this experience.

the focus on effective communication is critical for a clinical nurse at every level of licensure. Communication is one of the major leadership competencies defined by the American Nurses Association (2018). Within the concept of communication, "clear and concise writing" is an essential and necessary skill for all registered nurses (p. 7). The writing activities for registered nurses range from generating patient notes to cultivating treatment plans. The purpose of writing in the clinical environment is to be clear and effective, but nurses also have to choose words that most accurately reflect the situation (Lynn, 2019).

Obstacles From Clinical Experiences: Assumptions

Nurses write in the clinical setting on almost every shift. The landscape has shifted through the years, with more sophisticated electronic medical records, but the general tasks remain, including clinical notes, communication to providers, admission assessments, and discharge instructions. The nature of writing in the clinical environment can negatively impact nursing students through one main activity: making assumptions (meaning the reader understands the context of the written work).

First, clinical nurses assume the reader (other nurses, providers, ancillary staff, etc.) has access to the same information about the patient and uses the same general language within the clinical context. Nurses can refer to a particular lab result, and the reader can easily access the labs within the record. Additionally, nurses can refer to the inpatient psychiatric unit, and most of the readers do not need a detailed description of the furniture in the milieu. This streamlines the process for communication in the clinical environment. However, assuming the reader is well versed (as in the clinical setting) in scholarly writing can be detrimental. The results are poorly constructed arguments and research problems not having thorough, compelling descriptions.

Second, clinical nurses are well trained in giving specific facts about a patient or disease process. While this is extremely efficient when communicating about specific issues, problems arise in scholarly writing assignments. If students write in a similar fashion of only presenting facts or topics, their sentences may not connect or flow. The result is a lack of transition or argument development.

Third, grammatical and structurally sound writing is not a priority in clinical settings (especially during emergent situations). Though this is understandable in clinical situations, poor grammar can weaken any scholarly writing assignment. The result can be devastating for a grade.

Strengths From Clinical Experiences: Conciseness

The clinical setting can also have a positive effect on nurses engaging in scholarly writing. Nurses are concise and can quickly get to the point. Graduate students in other disciplines may struggle by writing with too many descriptive terms and may lack having a target to their writing, whereas nurses are well skilled at focusing on their point. More detail of conciseness, clarity, and precision are included in Chapter 3.

A second positive effect from clinical experiences is that nurses can articulate why certain disease processes are important. They do this naturally when talking with patients, and most have the skills to explain to a patient or caregiver the level of seriousness of a particular disease. Nurses take time in carefully describing a disease process and clinical implications. They may use metaphors or emotional language to connect with patients or caregivers. Nurses may also alter their language to meet patients or caregivers of various health literacy levels. These same skills are directly applicable to scholarly writing. Graduate nursing students can write clearly and effectively just as efficiently as when communicating with patients.

In summary, writing in clinical settings may have a negative impact on scholarly writing, and graduate students should be aware of this tension. However, several positive effects from clinical experiences can also benefit graduate students' writing. Distinguishing between the skills needed for each type of writing and carefully applying the accompanying rules are critical for success in graduate school.

If you already see a tension between what you experience in the clinical setting versus the feedback you receive on your academic assignments, do not worry; this is normal. This workbook is designed to be a guide and provide a means to bridge these worlds.

References

American Nurses Association. (2018). *Competency model.* https://www.nursingworld.org/~4a0a2e/globalassets/docs/ce/177626-ana-leadership-booklet-new-final.pdf

Butcher, J. N. (2009). *Clinical personality assessment: History, evolution, contemporary models, and practical applications.* https://doi.org/10.1093/oxfordhb/9780195366877.013.0001

Carnevale, A. P., Smith, N., Melton, M., & Price, E. W. (2015). Learning while earning: The new normal. Georgetown University Center on Education and the Workforce.

Dundes, L., & Marx, J. (2006). Balancing work and academics in college: Why do students working 10 to 19 hours per week excel? *Journal of College Student Retention: Research, Theory & Practice, 8*(1), 107–120. https://doi.org/10.2190/7UCU-8F9M-94QG-5WWQ

Edmunds, M. W., & Waldrop, J. (2018). What is scholarly writing? *The Journal for Nurse Practitioners, 14*(8), A11–A12. https://doi.org/10.1016/j.nurpra.2018.08.012

Fonseca, J. R. F. d., Calache, A. L. S. C., Santos, M. R. d., Silva, R. M. d., & Moretto, S. A. (2019). Association of stress factors and depressive symptoms with the academic performance of nursing students. *Revista da Escola de Enfermagem da USP, 53*, 1–9. https://doi.org/10.1590/S1980-220X2018030403530

Haghbin, M., McCaffrey, A., & Pychyl, T. A. (2012). The complexity of the relation between fear of failure and procrastination. *Journal of Rational-Emotive & Cognitive-Behavior Therapy, 30*(4), 249–263. https://doi.org/10.1007/s10942-012-0153-9

Horning, A. S. (1987). *Teaching writing as a second language.* Southern Illinois University Press.

Krashen, S. D. (1982). *Principles and practice in second language acquisition.* Prentice-Hall. https://books.google.com/books?id=LRFZAAAAMAAJ

Llego, J., Gabriel, E., & Corpus, J. (2018). A correlational study on the stress level and academic performance of nursing students. *Journal of Basic and Applied Research, 4*(4), 83–87.

Lynn, P. B. (2019). *Taylor's clinical nursing skills: A nursing process* (5th ed.). Wolters Kluwer.

Micsinszki, S. K., & Yeung, L. (2021). Adapting "Shut Up & Write!®" to foster productive scholarly writing in graduate nursing students. *The Journal of Continuing Education in Nursing, 52*(7), 313–318. http://ddoi.org/10.3928/00220124-20210611-05

National Institute of Mental Health. (2018). *Anxiety disorders.* https://www.nimh.nih.gov/health/topics/anxiety-disorders

Penn, J. (2016). *The successful author mindset: A handbook for surviving the writer's journey.* Amazon KDP.

Pike, G. R., Kuh, G. D., & Massa-McKinley, R. C. (2008). First-year students' employment, engagement, and academic achievement: Untangling the relationship between work and grades. *NASPA Journal, 45*(4), 560-582. https://doi.org/10.2202/1949-6605.2011

Rocha Cesar, F. C., Teixeira Sousa, E., Miranda Ribeiro, L. C., & de Almeida Cavalcante Oliveira, L. M. (2018). Graduate school stressors: An integrative literature review. *Cogitare Enfermagem, 23*(4), 86–96. https://doi.org/10.5380/ce.v23i4.57460

Silvia, P. J. (2019). *How to write a lot: A practical guide to productive academic writing* (2nd ed.). American Psychological Association. https://doi.org/10.1037/0000109-000

Wynne, C., Guo, Y.-J., & Wang, S.-C. (2014). Writing anxiety groups: A creative approach for graduate students. *Journal of Creativity in Mental Health, 9*(3), 366–379. https://doi.org/10.1080/15401383.2014.902343

CHAPTER 2

Types of Audiences

Pearman D. Parker and Elizabeth Riley

We define "audience" as your reader. This can range from a faculty member to a peer or trusted friend, to a national committee of nurses. Regardless of the details of your audience, your job is to convince them of your position and your work.

Upon embarking on your writing assignment, the first thing you want to do is orient your audience to your topic. You cannot assume the reader is as well versed in a clinical problem as you are. Similarly, you cannot assume that your reader knows anything about your nursing specialty. The key is to use this assumption to your advantage. Ideally you want to convince the reader of your credibility, and that your words warrant the audience's time. Your responsibility is to walk the reader through your ideas in a carefully constructed manner. You should write with conviction and purpose, and include evidence for your argument (data, interpretation, references to other scholarly work) to develop the reader's credibility toward your position (and your writing).

Nurses are generally quite skilled in convincing their clinical audience (i.e., the patient) to engage them in some specific behavior. For example, a nurse may need to educate a patient about a new oral medication for diabetes. The nurse must communicate in such a way that the patient is convinced of the importance of taking the prescribed medication to control diabetes. Generally, this involves the nurse first taking an initial assessment regarding the patient's existing knowledge about diabetes followed by an individualized educational session regarding the medication. Nurses must assess an individual's baseline knowledge and then provide tailored education specific to the patient (Lowenstein & Bradshaw, 2004). Perhaps this patient has mentioned to the nurse that they are a devoted grandparent and loves spending time with their grandchildren but found recent interruptions in playtime. The nurse may use this knowledge to educate the patient about the benefits of controlling diabetes. See the following script:

> I know you mentioned earlier that you have episodes of dizziness, sweating, and shakiness that can interfere with playtime with the grandkids. Did you know, according to the American Diabetes Association, that these are signs of a hypoglycemic episode? Evidence shows that taking your newly prescribed medication for diabetes in conjunction with diet and exercise can help you have less of these hypoglycemic episodes. One benefit of this medication is that you may have more uninterrupted playtime with your grandkids.

Before moving any further with education or the when and why of the medication, the nurse has immediately gotten the attention of her audience (patient) and increased the likelihood that the patient will listen and comply with the treatment regimen by showcasing how the medication can help with an activity the patient enjoys. In addition, the nurse used evidence from the American Diabetes Association to add credibility to the information. In this scenario, the nurse could continue teaching the patient when and how often to take the medication, as well as about potential side effects using best evidence.

When your words are used correctly in the right combination, you as a writer can use this technique when considering your audience. Your goal is to write in such a way that you convince the audience of your position that what you have to say is worth their time and energy. Now that we have covered the overall approach to considering your audience, we offer you suggestions specific to each type of audience.

Faculty

While you are in graduate school, your faculty are your most important audience. You want to discern their expectations as quickly as possible to streamline your efforts. This can be hard for students, especially because faculty expectations can vary depending on the class, the specific assignment, and the faculty member's own expertise—not to mention their own comfort level with coaching students to write. Some faculty may be more concerned about your understanding of the content, while others may not assess the content until the grammar and structure is at a suitable level. We understand how frustrating this can be.

One remedy to this dilemma is to practice clarity in writing, and then the content will emerge. In addition, making strategic use the rubrics will be helpful with clarity and organizing your thoughts. On the other hand, if your writing lacks clarity, the content will not be conveyed.

Peers

Your peers may be your immediate classmates, other nursing graduate students at various points in their coursework or careers, or friends in other graduate programs. Generally, you have similar levels of experience and knowledge, and overall, you have one key aspect in common: You are all graduate students. We suggest that you use this to your advantage. You are all trying to learn how to write more clearly. You are all trying to craft compelling arguments to convince your audience (probably your faculty) about the worthiness of your written assignment.

Some faculty may ask you to have your peers read your work prior to submitting the assignment. This can be scary! Not only do you have the pressure to achieve a particular grade, but now you also want to make a good impression on your peers. Do not fall into this trap. If you are writing for your peers, try to remember what we emphasized in the beginning of this section: Write clearly; write with conviction; write with purpose. Your peers can be your biggest allies and strongest supporters. They may be the ones who encourage and motivate you when it seems like you cannot write one more word, let alone craft one more sentence. Since your peers can closely relate to your own struggles, they may also be gentler and more encouraging with feedback than the faculty may be. Additionally, do not discount the possible benefit of having peers from other disciplines read your work and offer feedback. They can offer valuable perspectives that you may not get to experience otherwise.

> I was struggling with one chapter in writing my dissertation. One of my committee members offered guidance, but in my mental and physical exhaustion, I was unable to receive her words and make the necessary revisions. Something was just not clicking. However, if I did not have the "aha" moment, my analysis would ultimately be flawed, and I would not have been able to pass my dissertation defense. I could imagine no worse outcome. I reached out to one of my peers in another field, and she read over the chapter that was causing me such torture. Somehow my peer was able to rephrase what my committee member had said and offered suggestions for next steps. The "aha" moment came rushing in full force. The mental lightbulb went on. The dissertation skies parted. To this day I remain forever indebted to the kindness of my peer. Even though she was in a totally different discipline, we were able to speak the same language. Sometimes reaching out to others can result in your greatest gifts.
>
> *Personal experience*, Pearman D. Parker, PhD, MPH, RN, PMH-BC

Nursing Colleagues

You may also write for an audience of nursing colleagues. For example, you might present your findings at local, state, or regional conferences. You may be asked to present results of a quality improvement project to hospital administrators. They may be more familiar with your specific nursing issue than your peers or faculty may be, but you must keep the same focus on clarity. Over the years, nursing has evolved from a skills-based discipline to a science (Pickler & Dorsey, 2022). Our predecessors in nursing were able to manage this transition at least partially thanks to their devotion to writing clear, concise information in a compelling way.

When you are writing for your nursing colleagues in a professional setting, you want to focus on the application of your findings. We call this the *so what* factor of your writing. For nursing, this often looks like patient-outcome indicators (financial, safety, infection rates, etc.).

You may not only need to take your audience through your clinical problem, but you may also need to present the answer with measurable outcomes. Let us use a clinical example to demonstrate what we mean.

Administrators in inpatient psychiatric settings often use seclusion and restraints as an outcome metric. As an administrator in this setting, you would create an evidence-based assessment tool for two main purposes. First, you want to identify patients at risk for violence toward staff. Second, you want to learn the best de-escalation strategies in advance of any aggressive behaviors. Your goal is to identify at-risk patients and have a plan in place to help de-escalate potential situations, thereby reducing the use of seclusion and restraints. Your *so what* factor here is that the tool will help decrease the use of seclusion and restraints (a primary outcome). When you present this clinical problem, assessment tool, and associated outcomes to your nursing colleagues, you will focus on clarity and conciseness. You have done a great deal of work and your writing needs to enhance the hard work you have already completed. Clear and explicit writing will showcase your hard work and your dedication to improving patient outcomes.

Nurses often have strong ideas that could lead to improved clinical outcomes (whatever those may be). However, sometimes nurses do not always have the skills to communicate their ideas. We want you to be in the best possible position by having the right attitude toward writing and the associated skills to be able to showcase your own clinical ideas.

In Summary

We hope to be your guide along your own writing journey with this workbook. We will use the next chapters to go through the details of the writing process. In Chapters 3 and 4, we will focus on the mechanics of grammar and organization. This will be focused on what we ourselves have seen from students, and we will offer suggestions to further refine your skills. We will then discuss useful strategies to avoid plagiarism in Chapter 5 by correctly incorporating scholarly literature and evidence into your writing. We will then shift from the mechanics of writing to deal with, and overcome, your negative emotions surrounding writing in Chapter 6. Lastly, Chapters 8 and 9 will focus on how to respond to criticism and will also discuss the delicate art of giving and responding to peer review.

References

Lowenstein, A. J., & Bradshaw, M. J. (2004). *Fuszard's innovative teaching strategies in nursing.* Jones & Bartlett Learning.

Pickler, R. H., & Dorsey, S. G. (2022). Shifting paradigms in nursing science. *Nursing Research, 71*(1), 1–2. https://doi.org/10.1097/NNR.0000000000000558

CHAPTER 3

Grammar

James V. Parker, Jr., Pearman D. Parker, and Elizabeth Riley

All good writing contains similar features: (a) a sense of purpose, (b) clarity, (c) excellent sentence structure and mechanics, and (d) a belief that the destination has been reached. Here, each of these areas will be presented in a manner that should be helpful as you become a scholarly writer.

What Is Writing?

Writing is a deliberate act that is undertaken to convey an idea, a feeling, a purpose, or a compilation of facts. Writing comes in all varieties—romantic writings such as poetry, philosophical writings expressing complex thinking, and informal writing, the most commonly used form of writing. Writing is one of our methods of communicating, and all methods share one characteristic: intent. Writing and other methods of communication are intentional acts directed toward an identified audience.

By example, writing and painting can be compared to demonstrate a deliberate act such as painting a house or a vehicle. The act is the same for both, but the method to complete each project is significantly different. This workbook is intended to help you to improve individual writing skills and your effectiveness as a writer.

Clarity and Precision

The effective writer must identify the audience. The writer must be able to articulate the purpose of the intentional act of writing. The writer must be able to convey their ideas with clarity and precision. Clarity is the state of being clear (Merriam-Webster, 2022a). Writing with clarity means that the reader understands exactly what the writer intends to convey. The other concept of precision is closely related. Precision is the state of being precise or accurate (Merriam-Webster, 2022b). Writing with precision means using as few words as possible to directly convey information (Bernstein, n.d.). These two concepts are interdependent. One must write precisely (meaning each word is carefully chosen) without sacrificing the clarity of the sentence. Clarity and precision are requisite to effective writing, and the physical structure of the written words can promote clarity and precision, but faulty mechanics (grammar and word choice) will surely undermine a writer's best efforts to write effectively.

Writing is a deliberate act that encourages a fluent use of words. The words that the writer uses create the wonderful colors that can be used to enhance the clarity of what the writer is trying to convey. The romantic writer, Alfred Noyes (1906), wrote this in his poem, "The Highwayman": "The moon was a ghostly galleon tossed upon cloudy seas" to describe the night in which one of his characters would appear. The word choice of "ghostly galleon" is called a metaphor. A philosophical writer, Descartes, simply said, "I think, therefore I am" to convey the notion that he existed because he could think (Descartes & Veitch, 1910). Both authors were reaching for clarity and precision and were successful through using different words, inferences, and thinking. In other words, there is more than one way to write with clarity and precision.

A WORD ON CLARITY Nursing students often struggle with clarity because they incorrectly assume the audience consists of other nurses who have the same basic understanding of their topic (e.g., disease process or population). This is likely the result of working in a clinical environment or on a unit in which other nurses share the same language and concepts about a particular topic. While this shared understanding allows nurses to practice more efficiently and safely, nursing students need to take additional efforts to ensure clarity prevails.

We recommend the following questions to check your clarity:

- Can this be interpreted any other way?
- Do these words mean what I think they mean?
- Would another nurse from another unit understand this?
- Does the sentence sound clear when I read it aloud?

We recommend the following strategies to correct for clarity:

- Look up meaning of words in a dictionary and use a thesaurus to see if any other words resonate better with you.
- Try breaking up a long sentence into two shorter sentences.
- Start off by writing "What I mean to say is . . ." as this will help to identify the point of the sentence. Once the point is identified, then go back and edit out the beginning. You should then be left with a straightforward sentence.

A WORD ON PRECISION Overall, nursing students with clinical experience excel at writing (and communicating) with precision. This is largely due to writing effective clinical notes and communicating efficiently with providers when the emphasis is to "get to the point." An example we like to use is picking the right needle gauge for an injection. A smaller needle is more precise and leaves less room for trauma. The same goes for scholarly writing: More precision means that your words will be less likely to be misunderstood. As you transition into writing scholarly papers, please remember this hidden strength of picking the right, precise needle gauge. You already have the skills to remove the clutter, or excess words, when editing your work.

Sample sentence:

- *You already have the skills to remove the clutter, or excess words, when editing your work.*

Sample sentence, but more precise:

- *You have the skills to remove excess words when editing.*

Active Voice

Clarity and precision can also be enhanced with active voice. Active voice is when the subject of the sentence is who or what performs an action of the verb (University of Chicago Press, 2017). Passive voice is used when "joining an inflected form of to be verbs with a verb's past participle" (p. 264). Active voice is regarded as more direct and vigorous, whereas passive voice is seen as less direct and less concise (Strunk & White, 1999). Active voice is recommended for scholarly writing and helps the writer to achieve clarity and precision.

A WORD ON ACTIVE VERSUS PASSIVE VOICE Active voice is a simple, yet easily forgotten concept in scholarly writing. The easiest way to think about active voice is that you want to clarify who is doing whatever action (or verb). You do not want to confuse your reader. Be careful reading the literature, as many publications are written in passive voice, and you may begin to emulate without necessarily noticing which voice you are using. Writing in active voice can take time to perfect and is most easily done when writing the initial drafts. It is much easier to write in active voice than trying to edit your work in passive voice.

Active voice:

- The nurse reconstituted the medication.
- A patient refused to take his nightly medication.

Passive voice:

- The medication was reconstituted.
- The medication was refused by the patient.

Fine-Tuning Grammar

Our goal here is to assist each writer in becoming more effective by identifying frequently incurred obstacles to effective writing that will be encountered along the way. The mechanical structure of writing, usually referred to as "grammar," can be a huge problem but can be overcome with patient practice. Each writer brings to class a unique writing experience with varying skill levels. Being willing to acknowledge one's own strengths and weaknesses will go a long way to minimize the negative effects related to grammatical areas of concern.

The primary areas of concern for grammatical issues are (a) sentence structure, (b) subject/verb agreement, (c) conjunctions and prepositions, (d) punctuation, and (e) phrases.

Sentence Structure

Sentence structure is much like the example of house painting. How the house is supposed to look after being painted is the same thing as how our writing is supposed to read when completed. Some of the house can be painted with large brush strokes, while other parts must be carefully touched up, and it is the same with writing. The writer should intend to write each sentence as they paint a room so that the outcome desired of having a beautifully decorated house will be realized.

Subject/Verb Agreement

Subject/verb agreement is when the subject of the sentence is singular (one of them) and the corresponding verb is also singular in form: "Mary is the president." Mary, the subject, is singular, and "is" the verb is also singular.

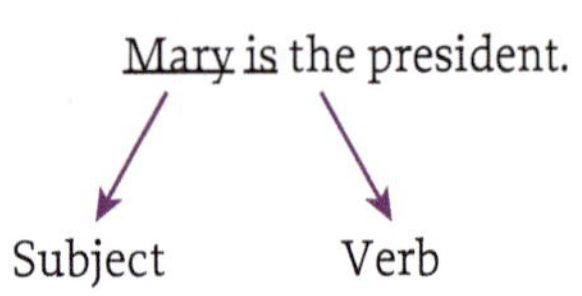

FIGURE 3.1 Subject/verb agreement.

This is the same for plural subjects and plural verbs. Examples of plural verbs are *are, use, run, were* (with exceptions), *see*. None of these verbs ends in "s." Look at the previous sentence. "None" is the singular subject and "ends" is a singular verb. Do not get detoured by the prepositional phrase in the middle, "of these verbs." Verbs is plural but not the subject. The "fix" for this is to be sure what the subject is and the requisite verb form. Knowing the subject should point to the correct verb choice.

The easiest way to identify many of these problems is to *read your sentence aloud*. Ask if the sentence conveys what was intended with clarity and precision. Ask if the subjects and verbs agree. If so, move on. If not, you want to go back to the drawing board of revisions. Sometimes a sentence may read correctly but not sound right. You may have a hard time identifying what the "issue" or "problem" with the sentence is, and in that case, simply revise until the sentence sounds correct.

Conjunctions and Prepositions

Conjunctions and prepositions cause frequent problems when used inappropriately. Use a dictionary or thesaurus to help identify what part of speech a word is. A conjunction is essentially any word that "connects sentences, clauses, or words within a clause" (University of Chicago Press, 2017, p. 287). If the word is a conjunction, do not use it to begin a sentence.

You will want to refrain from using these words at the beginning of sentences at all costs.

A preposition (or prepositional phrase) has an "an uninflected function word or phrase linking a noun element (the preposition's element) with another part of the sentence to show the relationship" (University of Chicago Press, 2017, p. 279). Essentially, prepositions give an indication of direction (in, around, near), position (above, behind), time (after, near), and the source (behind) of some object. Prepositional phrases, sometimes referred to as complex prepositions, include a preposition and a verb. An example prepositional phrase is "over the wood" and "through the woods" when referring to the direction to grandmother's house. Prepositions are fun to use but can be tricky. Remember to look for phrases when a preposition is encountered. It may be permissible to begin a sentence with a preposition, but a complete understanding of the "phrase" that follows is necessary to prevent faulty writing. Common prepositional phrases such as "over the hill" or "to the team" should not be used to begin a sentence. Frequently, prepositions are cliches and are not useful to clear writing. The problems such use can cause are not worth losing sentence effectiveness.

Examples of conjunctions:

- Simple: *and, but, if, or, though*
- Compound: *although, because, nevertheless, furthermore*

However (this is an introductory conjunction), infinitive phrases always begin with a preposition, and these phrases when used as a whole can act like a noun and be the subject of a sentence.

Here is such an example: "To dance is to live." "To dance" is the singular subject, and "is" is the singular verb. "To live" is another infinitive phrase acting as a noun.

These examples are also part of your overall sentence structures, which are intended to convey thoughts and ideas with clarity and precision. The word choices affect the end result of every written document.

Examples of prepositions:

- Simple preposition: *at, by*
- Compound preposition: *into, outside, upon*

Examples of prepositional phrases:

- *according to*
- *by means of*
- *with regard to*

Independent and Dependent Clauses

Another common obstacle for the writer is knowing the difference between an independent clause and a dependent clause. A clause is more developed than a simple prepositional phrase. Independent clauses have a subject and a verb, and the independent clause can stand alone as a sentence. For example, "Mary is the president, and Jane is the treasurer." "Mary is the president" is one independent clause, and "Jane is the treasurer" is another independent clause. Both have a subject and a verb and can stand alone if separated.

Dependent clauses, however, *cannot* stand alone as a sentence. Dependent clauses depend on other parts of the sentence to give them support and meaning. An example of this is, "Mary, the president of General Stores, who is a millionaire." The example is dependent because it has no corresponding verb to give it support. "Is" is a verb in the clause, but "who" is the subject of that phrase. Identifying the difference between independent clauses and dependent clauses will save the writer time when editing. Writing with clarity and precision always requires editing to obtain the most effective outcome.

Commas

Finally, the proper use of the comma will be ever present in writing efforts. Generally, the writer should always be aware of where the subject is placed in the sentence and where the corresponding verb is located. The term *comma splice* is used when a comma has been inappropriately placed between the subject(s) and the verb(s).

Please note that comma splices are easy to create when using them to signal a pause in speech. Pausing while speaking can be an effective technique in communicating, but you need to make sure that your written word is correct.

Consult a grammar book when questions about comma placement or use arise. Regardless of the grammatical or technical writing element in question, we recommend nursing students use outside writing resources to strengthen writing skills and learn the reasons for certain mechanics not currently explored here. We recommend using the Strunk and White (1999) book, *The Elements of Style*, as this is one of the most popular resources for writers regardless of their discipline. The two other resources are the most current editions of *The Chicago Manual of Style* and of the *Publication Manual of the American Psychological Association*. Nursing students generally see these resources as style manuals, but they also offer comprehensive direction for grammar, content, and how to avoid biased language.

Please note that we are offering suggestions to help you to become a more well-rounded writer with the appropriate knowledge and skills of the mechanics of writing. These books are to supplement whatever your professors or instructors recommend. We insist that you follow the style manual endorsed by your faculty first.

Picking the Right Words

A dictionary and a thesaurus are excellent sources for selecting the proper word that will be most effective to the reader. Dictionaries usually provide correct spelling, definitions, and some synonyms. A thesaurus will provide synonyms and definitions and suggest appropriate usage. Selecting the proper words is directly related to how well you know your audience and their expectations. Do not conclude, however, that your effectiveness will improve with the size of the word. "Big" words are only useful if three things exist: (a) The writer knows what the word means; (b) the audience knows what the word means in its context; and (c) the "big" word enhances clarity and precision.

Problem word choices are encountered frequently, and in virtually every instance, it is because the writer does not know the meaning or definition of the word chosen. The mechanics of English can be tricky. Competing sounds are often the problem as in "vise" and "advise" and "vice" and "advice." "Vise" and "vice" sound alike (homonyms) but are not the same. "Vise" and "vice" in "advice" also sound alike but are not the same. "Advise" is a verb. "Advice" is a noun. Another example for consideration is "affect" and "effect." "Effect" is typically a noun, and "affect" is typically a verb. Do not confuse the two. The thesaurus should help discern these pairs of apparently confusing words. Relying on the spell-check tool within common programs like Word or Pages will not catch these errors.

Take to heart the notion that effective writing is an intentional and deliberate act to convey an ideas, feelings, and facts with clarity and precision. Choose every word wisely.

Please note that choosing the right word often requires a level of attention and energy that sometimes alludes graduate nursing students. Many students know the difference between effect and affect but may use them incorrectly when tired. We recommend that editing and revising be done when you are more energized and can pay attention to details.

Several words that should be avoided in writing or speaking are *myself, himself, herself, themselves*, and *ourselves*. Give some thought to these words, which are chosen because the speaker or writer thinks they are stronger. In fact, these words are very weak and redundant. Keeping clarity and precision at the forefront eliminates redundancy in all forms. The adage "say what you mean, and mean what you say" applies here. "I did it myself" should be written as "I did it." The addition of "self" at the end of a word rarely, if ever, adds to clarity or precision.

One of the very best sources for word choice may be found by looking at a vintage, printed issue of *Reader's Digest* in the section entitled, "It Pays to Increase Your Word Power." Each month, 20 words are featured, with questions involving definitions, differences (advise, advice), and usage. Hundreds of examples of word choice issues can be found within the pages. *Reader's Digest* (2022) also offer online quizzes of different categories of quizzes from book-related words to words with double letters. Additionally, games such as Scrabble and *The New York Times* crossword puzzle are fun ways to strengthen your vocabulary and add enjoyment to your learning.

Conclusion

The deliberate act of writing requires a process of refining what has been written. Take the time to read aloud, loudly, if necessary, each paragraph before submitting it for review. This one act will improve the final draft for the clarity and precision desired. Stay away from using first and second person as subjects (I, me, you, they). This may be permissible for informal writing but rarely for writing for professional journals or for class assignments. Check with your instructor for guidance about this.

Revise! Revise! Revise!

Editing what is written before it is submitted for review or grading is necessary to improve clarity and precision. Plus, you may find new concepts/ideas or view things differently after you edit and revise. The simple act of revising can help you learn and think about topics in a different manner. In other words, editing can help the "light bulb go on."

Writing comes easy to some and not so much to others. As simple as it sounds, practice can make perfect, but the practice must be positive practice. When problems arise, as they do for all writers, seek other opinions from peers, your professors, and resource books. Think through the topic or issue at length and then draft an outline. Begin the intentional act of writing by choosing the words that will add color to your thoughts and ideas. When you encounter writing obstacles, seek assistance. Most of these issues at this stage can be corrected with a little diligence and practice.

Each college or university offers various levels of assistance. Some programs may offer intensive writing workshops whereas others may offer tutoring services through the library. Some faculty may offer to read initial drafts to provide feedback for both the quality and content of your writing. Generally, faculty will often make recommendations, or the college will endorse certain services. You can decide which one to try first. You may have to try several resources before finding one that fits for your style of writing and learning, but you can receive individual attention needed to refine your mechanics, word choice, and grammar.

References

Bernstein, D. S. (n.d.). *Precision writing.* University of Michigan. http://www-personal.umich.edu/~dsbaero/tutorials/PrecisionWritingV8.pdf

Descartes, R., & Veitch, J. (1910). *Discourse on the method of rightly conducting reason, and seeking truth in the sciences.* Open Court Publishing Company.

Merriam-Webster. (2022a). *Clarity.* https://www.merriam-webster.com/dictionary/clarity

Merriam-Webster. (2022b). *Precision.* https://www.merriam-webster.com/dictionary/precision

Noyes, A. (1906). The highwayman. *Blackwood's Magazine,* 244–247.

Reader's Digest. (2022). *Word power vocabulary quizzes.* https://www.rd.com/article/word-power/

Strunk, W., & White, E. B. (1999). *The elements of style* (4th ed.). Penguin.

University of Chicago Press. (2017). *The Chicago manual of style* (17th ed.). The University of Chicago Press.

Credit

CHAPTER 4

Organization

Pearman D. Parker and Elizabeth Riley

This chapter aims to introduce the concept of organization and teach you the skills needed to write in a logical, structured, and compelling manner.

What Is Organization?

One of the major weaknesses identified in student papers is organization. Faculty may use this term loosely, but conveying the exact definition can be difficult for students to understand. Essentially, organization in writing is the structure needed to convey a compelling argument. Organization is the framework needed to clarify ideas, link concepts, and persuade the reader. We conceptualize organization as the sentences, paragraphs, and sections in manuscripts. Without strong organization, the reader is often left feeling confused, lost, and unsure of the purpose of writing. Thus, organization is a critical (and sometimes overlooked) aspect of writing that all graduate nursing students must master in their scholarly writing.

As we touched on in previous chapters (see Chapters 2 – 3), every piece of writing should be conveyed in a compelling way. At the end of the written piece, the reader should believe the words and the argument and essentially have faith in the author's credibility. In other words, a compelling piece of writing means the reader is convinced of the writer's position. One of the best methods to persuade the reader is to strategically use sentences, paragraphs, and sections of the paper to convey the intended purpose. Plus, organization helps the writer, too. A well-organized document saves time, energy, and effort by helping you, the writer, communicate clearly and effectively.

Graduate nursing students may not think they have much experience writing in an organized fashion but have significant skills that can be applied to scholarly writing. Let's take the example of calling a physician or giving report to another nurse. Clinical nurses quickly identify the most crucial information and convey it in such a way that draws attention. Patient status and pertinent observations are disclosed upfront. Any questions are saved for the end of the conversation. This is done with careful organization—and shows that you (the one giving report or calling) have done your research and thought critically about the patient.

As you continue to refine your writing throughout your graduate school program, remember your ease with such clinical skills, as these same talents will transfer to writing, too. You have more skills than you may realize.

Terms

- Flow—The connection between ideas and thoughts; transitions between paragraphs.
  - Opposite: disjointed
- Linking—Connection of ideas to one another.
  - Opposite: jumping all around
- Fluid—How smoothly your sentences (and ideas) flow.
  - Opposite: choppy

How to Get Organized

Essentially only two steps exist in getting organized. The first step to writing in an organized fashion is to determine the purpose. The body (or sections) of the paper change depending on the assignment. The second step is to draft an outline (which we will describe in detail). The outline will contain the main points and references (when applicable). Staying focused on the purpose and constructing a solid outline are the two main components to writing in an organized way.

Starting With the Basics: Paragraphs

A paragraph is essentially a structured, organized set of sentences grouped together for one purpose. A paragraph may be large and conceptual or can be extremely detailed depending on the purpose for the paragraph. Some paragraphs are written in about two to three sentences, whereas other paragraphs can include several sentences. The paragraph may be a simple introduction to an idea or topic. A paragraph could also be written as a descriptive piece (e.g., to describe the effect of a specific disease process) or as a discussion section in which the writer presents various levels of evidence (e.g., presenting different results from similar studies).

A paragraph most always includes a topic sentence. The sentences that follow support the topic sentence or provide additional detail. The concluding sentence usually prepares the reader for a transition to the next paragraph or section in a paper. Ideally, you want to get into a flow (meaning an ease of conveying the meaning) between sentences.

Please note that writing sentences with a solid flow, linking one sentence to the next, reads easily. This does not mean that the task of doing so is easy. The product will read as if it was easy; this is good! Think of this like getting a good stick for an IV. Some nurses can make sticking an IV look incredibly easy, whereas others' hands shake the entire time. Do not get caught up in the emotions (as in frustration) of the process; the end result will read easily.

A strong sample paragraph will read as follows:

- Topic sentence to the paragraph
- Supporting sentence 1
- Supporting sentence 2
- Supporting sentence 3
- Conclusion

Working With an Example: The Perfect Vacation

We have found that teaching writing basics to graduate nursing students is most easily accomplished by using metaphors. For this exercise, let's take the example of a perfect vacation. *Please take a few minutes to think about your perfect vacation. You are welcome to jot down where you want to go and why this place would be your perfect vacation.*

____

____

____

____

Perfect Vacation Example: Not so Good

- I used to take family vacations all the time growing up. Vacations can be necessary to help with stress. I would like to go on a vacation. But I don't know where I would go. My folks used to take me to the beach. I want to go to the beach. That sounds fun.

Here is an example of a not-so-good paragraph response to a perfect vacation. Let's start off by talking about grammar. This writer switches tenses and leaves the reader confused. *(We advise you to only use one tense per paragraph.)* The first sentence reads as if the writer will talk about family vacations—a nostalgic opening sentence. However, then the writer jumps to present and future tense. Midway through the paragraph the writer goes back to past tense before concluding that a beach trip would be fun. In terms of content, this paragraph reads like a stream of consciousness and appears disjointed. The reader is also unclear about the main point of the paragraph. Was the writer talking about a vacation? A need for a beach trip? The purpose of remembering childhood vacations? Without clear, organized sentences the reader cannot stay on track with the purpose of the paragraph.

Perfect Vacation Example: Good

- My idea of a perfect vacation would be a week-long stay at an island in the Caribbean. I would relax by the blue waters and enjoy the fresh flowers around me. The waves would give a calming sound. The breeze would gently brush through my hair. The sand between my toes will feel like little exfoliating rocks. I will be at peace without a care in the world. That would be my idea of the perfect vacation.

This is an example of a good paragraph. The topic sentence opens the paragraph and sets the stage. The reader knows immediately that the focus is an ideal vacation in the Caribbean, which has yet to happen (pay attention to the verb tense here). Each sentence thereafter supports the topic sentence. The supportive sentences touch on water, flowers, waves, breezes, and sand. By the end of the paragraph, the reader has several compelling reasons to believe the writer's perspective that an island in the Caribbean would be a perfect vacation.

Please note that when reading others' work (or editing your own) the goal is not to necessarily agree with the topic or position of the paragraph. Not everyone likes beaches, heat, and sand. Instead, the goal is to provide evidence (or reasons) that support the writer's position. Basically, the question here is: Do I (the reader) believe that this is the writer's version of a perfect vacation? The same question can be applied in scholarly writing, although we write with more evidence and less opinion.

Perfect Vacation Example: Best

- I want to be transported to the magical world of Paris for the perfect vacation. The glimmering city lights will ignite a sparkle in my soul. The bewitching art galleries will dance in my eyes. The whispers of the ancient artifacts will sing to me tales of the past. Every day and every night will be filled with a unique combination of adventure and stillness. The enchantment of Paris will forever be my perfect vacation to restore my heart and my soul.

The writer of this particular paragraph has one goal: Convince the reader that a vacation in Paris is perfect. The topic sentence sets the stage of Paris. The writer then uses each sentence to not only describe a facet of the vacation but also to convey the effect this has on the writer. As a result, each sentence has a good deal of context beyond just a descriptive piece. Lastly, the writer wraps up the paragraph with the concluding sentence, tying together a neatly packaged paragraph.

Please note that the Paris sentences are heavy in context; you want to aim for this in scholarly writing. You present evidence and then describe the impact (or influence, association, etc.) on your topic (patient population, disease process, etc.).

Applying Your Clinical Skills

The next step in learning how to write a well-crafted paragraph is to apply clinical skills. We will now move away from the perfect vacation scenario and use a nurse's note. Clinical nurses write a nurse's note each shift and focus on descriptive terms, observations, and facts to document a patient's condition. While nurses' notes are not equivalent to a scholarly paragraph, simple adjustments in thought processes can help graduate nursing students compose well-written paragraphs.

Table 4.1 is an exercise in which we take a nurse's note on a patient with heart failure and transition the topic of heart failure into a scholarly paragraph.

TABLE 4.1 Nurse's Notes Versus Scholarly Paragraph

Nurse's Note	Thought Process	Scholarly Paragraph
Crackles in lower lobes bilaterally. Skin color dusky. No signs of respiratory distress noted. No persistent cough noted. Lower extremities pitting 4+ edema. Patient's weight remained the same. Spouse visited patient today. Call light within reach and fall precautions initiated.	How do I take a patient's clinical experience and write a scholarly paragraph? *Focus on the broad concept of heart failure and how it applies to many patients.* How do I get my reader to believe the information being presented? *Clinical nurses rely on their clinical expertise and observation as evidence. When writing scholarly paragraphs, the evidence becomes other people's work, which you must cite. It is not enough to simply reply on your own observations or clinical experience for scholarly work.*	Heart failure is ___ (define) (cite American Heart Association). This chronic disease affects approximately ___% men and ___% women in the United States annually. The signs and symptoms of uncontrolled heart failure include pulmonary edema, shortness of breath, and poor perfusion, all of which lead to increased morbidity and mortality.
Rationale and compelling evidence: A nurse's note is written with incomplete sentences. The goal is to briefly and succinctly convey information about the patient's status. The evidence given is the nurse's assessment findings and any changes noted.		**Rationale and compelling evidence:** The purpose of the scholarly paragraph is to describe the importance of heart failure using evidence. The clinical symptoms written in the nurses' note are also conveyed here.

Pay particular attention to the middle column of the two main questions. First, you need to ask yourself how you can take a clinical topic and present the topic in a scholarly manner. Many graduate nursing students (and even faculty) experience difficulty in thinking about a patient problem on a larger scale. This is normal. Do not be dismayed! Second, you want to think about the evidence you need to support your paragraph. Evidence for a scholarly paragraph includes facts, statistics, and research findings.

Moving Beyond One Paragraph

Building the body of a paper can be overwhelming, but the same structure for each paragraph remains the same. Instead of focusing on just one paragraph to support a point, the writer will string together several connected paragraphs to reinforce the purpose. When writing larger papers (or assignments), graduate nursing students can sometimes face challenges staying focused on their overall message (or purpose). We recommend using an outline to keep the paragraphs connected to support the purpose.

What Is an Outline?

An outline is the framework for your paper or larger scholarly writing assignment. A strong outline allows the writer to connect paragraphs and topics throughout a paper. In other words, an outline is the structure that holds paragraphs. More frequently, outlines are used for papers with several paragraphs (greater than 2 pages), but outlines can be used for smaller assignments (less than 2 pages), as the concepts are transferrable.

A basic outline consists of an introduction, main topics, and a conclusion. Each heading (seen as "Topic") consists of supporting evidence. Each level of supporting evidence can be written as one stand-alone sentence or threaded together using conjunctions and complex sentences (see Chapter 3). A basic outline is as follows:

1. Introduction
    a. Main point 1
    b. Main point 2
    c. Main point 3
    d. Purpose
2. Topic 1
    a. Supporting evidence 1.1
    b. Supporting evidence 1.2
    c. Supporting evidence 1.3
3. Topic 2
    a. Supporting evidence 2.1
    b. Supporting evidence 2.2
    c. Supporting evidence 2.3
4. Conclusion

Sample Outlines

The basic structure of outlines is useful regardless of the piece of scholarly writing. We present two main types of outlines that should be helpful in your graduate nursing school curriculum: the article critique and the research paper.

Please note that these are general suggestions for common assignments in graduate nursing school. We advise you to follow the rubric and set up your outline in accordance with it. This will help you stay focused and not waste energy or time.

Sample Article Critique Outline

An article critique is a written assignment with the purpose of not only summarizing a research article, but also evaluating the content of the article.

Content for this outline was adapted from the University of Arizona's (2021) Writing Center:

1. Introduction
    a. Overview of article
    b. Purpose of article critique

    Here you will write about one to two paragraphs introducing the article and purpose of the article.

2. Summary
    a. Purpose of research article (to explore, to describe, to measure an association, to test a theory, etc.)
    b. Methods used to answer research question
    c. Research findings

    In about two paragraphs you will describe the purpose, methods, and findings. The key here is to report only the facts. You want to stay aligned with your outline; otherwise, you may get lost in the writing.

3. Critique
    a. Strengths (ranging from purpose to research question, to methods, to results, to interpretations)

    Use your textbook resources to support your argument for why a particular point is a strength. Be as detailed as possible. You need to show your instructor that you can apply material learned in class for this critique.

    b. Weaknesses (ranging from purpose to research question, to methods, to results, to interpretations)

Use your textbook resources to support your argument for why a particular point is a weakness. Be specific about the weaknesses. You may also want to draw on other concepts central to science (e.g., bias, sample size, etc.), as this will show your instructor your skills to apply material covered in and out of class. Hint: Some weaknesses are covered in the limitations section of the original article.

c. Assessment of article (believable, sound, rigor, etc.)

This can be a challenging area for students, so we recommend that you use the outline to assist not only writing but also your thought process. Take each section slowly, and discuss each area with intention. If you can build strong arguments for either the strengths or weaknesses, your assessment should flow naturally and logically.

4. Conclusion

a. Summary of key points and assessment

You want to tie this together in about four to five sentences. Try to write this as an overview summary. Stay broad, and do not repeat yourself verbatim. Instead, focus on large concepts.

Sample Research Paper Outline

Nursing graduate students will write a variety of research papers ranging from Doctorate of Nursing Practice to Doctor of Philosophy programs. We provide a general overview of using an outline. See other recommended resources for more detail (Grove et al., 2013):

I. Introduction (two to four paragraphs)

a. Background (statistics, rates, ratios, etc.)

You want to use relevant, up-to-date statistics to describe the problem for your population.

b. Presentation of research problem and review of relevant literature

Here, you can go into a bit more detail about the clinical problem or about your population. You may want to talk about the effect of the problem on groups of people, communities, health care systems, or national well-being. You should briefly mention relevant literature to your problem to provide the appropriate context for your paper. Nurses generally do well with this part; just remember to think about the problem beyond your one patient.

c. Purpose of research paper

Generally, the introduction is where you hook the reader. You will present a compelling argument for your clinical issue (or problem) and explicitly state why this topic needs to be investigated. Also, the introduction is an opportunity to give a good first impression, so be careful with your grammar and sentence structure. By the end of the introduction your reader should believe that your problem is definitely worthy of research and something the reader should care about (regardless if they actually do).

II. Methods

   a. Research design
   b. Setting
   c. Sampling

      i. Recruitment methods (if applicable)
      ii. Intended sample size (if applicable)

   d. Data collection

      i. Procedure

   Data collection can be tedious. A trick is keeping detailed notes during your research so you can easily write this section. Remember, you want to be clear and detailed so that your methods can be replicated.

   e. Analysis

      i. Type of analysis
      ii. Software used

   f. Other: Data safekeeping, institutional review board (IRB) approval

   Writers often begin their papers by writing the methods section first, which can be dry, boring, and detailed. Most critiques from peer review stem from writers not being clear enough in their methods.

III. Results

   a. Final sample size

   Here, you will talk about the process for reaching your final sample size. You will detail any missing data or lost data due to attrition.

   b. Specific results

   Your results are straightforward and leave little room for discussion or conjecture. You simply want to write what the results are in a narrative form.

IV. Discussion

   a. Interpretation of results

   You can now discuss your results by focusing on their implications. You want to take the reader through the logical application of your findings. Use each sentence as a building block to the next sentence.

b. Presentation of your results coupled with literature

After you interpret your results, you want to discuss your results in relation to the other literature. You can do this by comparing your findings with other research studies.

c. Speculation about your results (optional)

You may also want to expand on why your results appeared a certain way. You may see phrases like "we surmise" or "this could be due to . . .," and you want to walk the reader through your thought process.

d. Limitations

Use one paragraph to describe any limitations to your study. We recommend only writing three or four limitations. For each limitation you want to defend your research. For example, let's say you say had a small sample size in a qualitative study (~10 interviews) but reached data saturation (meaning no new data emerged, thus you could stop data collection). The limitation would read as such: "Our study is limited somewhat by our small sample size, but we reached data saturation and have confidence in our interpretation of the results."

V. Conclusion

a. State the conclusions of your research at addressing your problem

This is the last time you can convince your reader of the worthiness of your research question to address your problem. You can and should be broad here. You may be able to include recommendations for future studies or clinical implications (refer to the rubric or journal requirements). Please be careful with this section. Many students (and faculty) are tired by the end of the paper, and their writing reflects this. You want to end well.

A Final Note on Organization

Writing in an organized fashion takes time to refine. Much energy is expended up front to make an outline, but the result is worth the investment. A well-organized scholarly writing assignment demonstrates your ability to excel as a future nurse practitioner or scientist.

References

Grove, S. K., Burns, N., & Gray, J. R. (2013). Disseminating research findings. In *The practice of nursing research: Appraisal, synthesis, and generation of evidence* (7th ed.). Elsevier.

University of Arizona. (2021). *Writing an article critique.* https://writingcenter.uagc.edu/writing-article-critique

CHAPTER 5

Plagiarism and Paraphrasing

How to Avoid One and Do the Other

Elizabeth Riley and Pearman D. Parker

Plagiarism. This can easily be one of the most feared words used in graduate school. Almost every syllabus contains verbiage about plagiarism and consequences if students are suspected of it. Graduate nursing students may even begin to fear being suspected of plagiarism more than the actual act. We suspect that many graduate nursing students may not fully realize what plagiarism is or understand the various aspects of plagiarism. This is where we aim to help you. We will use this chapter to discuss the different types of plagiarism and include exercises to help you paraphrase correctly. Well-written paraphrasing is the ultimate way to protect yourself against plagiarism.

Plagiarism is defined as taking another's written work and using it as your own. This is an egregious act in general, but especially in academia, as this is similar to stealing another's thoughts and ideas. As a model graduate nursing student and registered nurse, this is definitely something you want to avoid. Similar to clinical work, your nurse's note is your own and not copied/pasted from another's note. This is particularly important for the legal weight that nurses' notes hold. Also, the nurse's note serves as evidence of your own clinical judgment regarding the patient. The same concepts can be applied for scholarly papers and assignments. The assignments represent your own thoughts and ideas around a particular issue (much like writing a progress note on a patient). However, a major difference between nurse's notes and scholarly assignments is that the content of scholarly papers is often borrowed from other scientific, scholarly papers (refer to Table 5.1). *Note: Scholarly papers are an integration of your own thoughts and ideas, coupled with other scholarly works. The key is to learn how to paraphrase the other sources so you can be free of plagiarism.*

TABLE 5.1 Examples of Sources Used in Scholarly Papers

Other Sources	Application to Scholarly Student Papers
Journal articles Books, book chapters	▪ Interventions in scientific studies ▪ Descriptive work captured in research studies ▪ Examples of case studies, quality improvement projects ▪ Other published statistics
Government sources	▪ Incidence, prevalence rates ▪ Odds ratios, hazard ratios ▪ Morbidity, mortality rates ▪ Population-level statistics

These multiple sources used within scholarly papers can be challenging to integrate into "your own words." Before we begin discussing how to paraphrase (and prevent plagiarism), we must first discuss the different categories of plagiarism.

Types of Plagiarism

The defined levels of plagiarism include direct plagiarism, mosaic plagiarism, and self-plagiarism (refer to Table 5.2). We define and give examples, as many people are not aware of different types of plagiarism.

TABLE 5.2 Types of Plagiarism

Type of Plagiarism	Definition	Example
Direct	"Word-for-word" use of someone else's writing without direct quotations, citation, and reference	Using a paragraph from a research article about the incidence of heart failure exactly as it reads, without direct quotes, citations, and reference; also known as the "copying and pasting"
Mosaic	Often referred to as "patch writing" or poor paraphrasing; occurs when certain words are replaced with synonyms and the sentence structure and overall thoughts are the same as previous author's	Writing a sentence from a textbook in the same structure and replacing three words with synonyms
Self	Using previous work for a current or future assignment without approval from both previous and current professors	Submitting a theoretical analysis paper from a previous nursing theory course to a current course without approval from both professors

Awareness of plagiarism is the first key to ensuring writers use their own words and thoughts, and use direct quotations for those particular phrases that have been worded "just right" by the previous author. The second key to prevent plagiarism is the use of well-written paraphrasing, which includes interpreting the previous author's work and expounding on that information into your own words. *Note: The best way to describe the process of paraphrasing is taking the gist of another's work and rewriting with the same gist in mind.*

This is not simply finding synonyms to replace a few words in the author's sentence (see Table 5.2 for mosaic plagiarism). Authors who effectively paraphrase and cite previous authors not only maintain writing integrity but are also much more likely to fully understand and grasp the concept they are writing about. There are several online sources to help with effective and good paraphrasing practices (see Table 5.3).

TABLE 5.3 Resources for Paraphrasing

Resources: Paraphrasing and Plagiarism
https://quillbot.com/guides/paraphrasing
https://owl.purdue.edu/owl/research_and_citation/using_research/quoting_paraphrasing_and_summarizing/paraphrasing.html
https://www.bowdoin.edu/dean-of-students/conduct-review-board/academic-honesty-and-plagiarism/examples.html
https://www.ox.ac.uk/students/academic/guidance/skills/plagiarism

Samples of Paraphrasing and Original Sources

See the following examples for mosaic plagiarism, poor paraphrasing, and good paraphrasing.

- *The yellow highlight represents the major concepts of the original source, which will need to be emphasized for quality paraphrasing. We recommend students to do the same with their original sources. Find the main points and write your own words off the main points.*

Sample 1

Original: An interactive, self-driven tutorial offered in an online format proved beneficial to adult students enrolled in the fully online, RN-BSN completion program at the study site (Riley, 2018).

Mosaic plagiarism/poor paraphrasing: An interactive, self-paced tutorial provided in a virtual format proved helpful to adult students completing a fully online, RN-BSN completion program (Riley, 2018).

- *This is too similar to the original source. Within the first few words of "interactive, self-paced tutorial" the faculty member is already suspicious. Some of the words changed, such as "proved helpful" instead of "proved beneficial," but work still needs to be done. This is where most graduate nursing students struggle. Remember, you want to retain the main points, but otherwise write from your own voice.*

Good paraphrasing: RN-BSN students may learn scholarly writing more effectively when the concepts of adult learning theory are used, specifically interactivity and self-pacing (Riley, 2018).

- *First, pay attention to how the order of the concepts has flipped. The start of the sentence is now about the type of student, and the specifics of the tutorial are listed last. Second, the author clearly understands that "more beneficial" and "more effective" are the same in this context. This type of well-written paraphrasing takes a little bit of time to really identify the main messages before crafting as your own.*

Sample 2

Original: In the US in 2022, an estimated 287,850 new cases of invasive breast cancer will be diagnosed among women and 43,250 women will die from the disease (American Cancer Society, 2022, p. 3).

- *Reminder: The highlighted areas represent the main points that can be carried over into your writing.*

For population statistics, double-check if the sentence you are citing has an additional reference. If no reference is cited, then you will cite the source you are using (e.g., American Cancer Society). If the sentence has a reference, cite that particular reference (usually listed under in the References section).

Mosaic plagiarism/poor paraphrasing: In the United States, about 287,850 women are diagnosed with invasive breast cancer yearly and 43,250 are estimated to die from breast cancer (American Cancer Society, 2022).

- *Faculty see this as a common issue when quoting population statistics. It reads too similarly to the original source. The format of the sentence is the same, and too few words were changed. You are allowed to be creative while keeping the same central information (highlighted).*

Good paraphrasing: More than 287,850 women are diagnosed with invasive breast cancer annually in the United States. Slightly more than 6% of these women (43,250) will die as a result from the same disease (American Cancer Society, 2022).

- *This is a bit more of a creative approach to the original source. First, the reference is split into two sentences. Second, including the 6% was for variety to the sentence but also maintained the same numbers. These skills do take time to develop, and a good bit of thinking is involved to accurately (and creatively) paraphrase with clear, effective writing.*

Practicing Paraphrasing Worksheet

Use the examples provided to practice your paraphrasing skills. Refer to the highlighted areas to identify the main points of the sentence.

Item 1

The results of the study show that an online tutorial for scholarly writing can be effective if highly structured, but also flexible for student participation, allowing students the opportunity to participate at a time and place of their choosing. Flexibility in participation relates to Knowles's adult learning theory and shows RN-BSN students can be successful in scholarly writing with the use of a tutorial when structured around Knowles's six assumptions of adult learners (Riley, 2018).

____

____

____

____

____

Item 2

An interactive, self-driven tutorial offered in an online format proved beneficial to adult students enrolled in the fully online, RN-BSN completion program at the study site. While many previous studies have researched the benefits of online tutorials, few studies exist with the use of an interactive scholarly writing tutorial specifically for RN-BSN students using a quantitative design. A tutorial that is interactive, structured, and self-paced offers adult learners flexibility and caters to their self-motivation while following the concepts of general tutoring by providing clear and concise learning material in a structured manner (Riley, 2018).

____

____

____

____

____

Item 3

A Mann-Whitney U test (Figure A) revealed a statistically significant difference in the median spelling and grammar rubric scores of RN-BSN nursing students between the pre-intervention (MD = 4.4, *n = 108) and post-intervention groups (MD = 4.75, n = 56), U = 2471, z = –1.95, p =.03, r = 0.15). A Mann-Whitney U test (Figure A) revealed a statistically significant difference in the median APA style rubric scores of RN-BSN nursing students between the pre-intervention (MD = 3.54, n = 108) and post-intervention groups (MD = 4.0, n = 56, U = 2616, z = –1.43, p = .02, r =0.11). A p value of < .05 indicates the null hypothesis is rejected. The use of an online scholarly writing tutorial impacted rubric scores (spelling and grammar, and APA style) when comparing a pre-intervention to a post-intervention group* (Riley, 2018).

____

____

____

____

____

Note: Including statistics can be challenging with paraphrasing. We generally recommend graduate nursing students include the means and p-values. If you are writing about more specific results of individual tests, then you can use the accompanying statistical results. Be sure to provide a reference at the end of your paragraph.

References

American Cancer Society. (2022). *Breast cancer facts & figures 2022-2024.* https://www.cancer.org/content/dam/cancer-org/research/cancer-facts-and-statistics/breast-cancer-facts-and-figures/2022-2024-breast-cancer-fact-figures-acs.pdf

Riley, E. (2018). *The impact of an online scholarly writing tutorial for RN-BSN students. SSRN.* https://doi.org/https://dx.doi.org/10.2139/ssrn.3238896

CHAPTER 6

Identifying and Reframing Emotions Associated With Writing

Pearman D. Parker and Elizabeth Riley

Do the thing you fear most and the death of fear is certain

—Mark Twain

... but was Mark Twain a nurse in graduate school?

A significant amount of pages in this book have been dedicated to the writing process. We covered topics such as organization, grammar, and outlines. The content has mostly focused on the energy, time, and skills needed to achieve the primary goal of composing a scholarly paper. While the tasks, skills, and effort put toward writing a scholarly paper are all valuable endeavors, students must also learn how to manage another component in writing: emotions.

The emotional responses associated with the writing process were briefly described in Chapter 1, and we offered a self-inventory to help graduate nursing students identify some of these emotions and the impacts on their writing.

In this chapter we will address the emotions surrounding writing more thoroughly. We will first discuss some frequent emotions associated with scholarly writing experienced by graduate nursing students and also describe the cultural narrative around writing. Next, we will discuss the emotions surrounding the lack of interest and experiences in clinical practice. We will conclude the chapter by discussing the commonly occurring concept of imposter syndrome and how this impacts scholarly writing both in school and in professional settings. Each of these sections will emphasize the importance of identifying emotions and reframing associated thoughts.

Please note that our goal is not for you to diminish your emotions surrounding writing. Instead, we want you to become more aware of your emotions toward writing so you can best navigate your own internal world. Ultimately, we want you to work with and manage your emotions of writing instead of fighting and resisting writing revisions or critical feedback.

Allowing Emotions With the Writing Process

The writing process includes a range of activities, from brainstorming ideas to outlining, to generating words and revising said words. Each of these activities can elicit different emotions at various times depending on your physical and internal environment (i.e., stress, mental health, emotional and physical wellness, etc.). Similarly, emotions may change depending on your own levels of writing self-efficacy (i.e., how much you believe in yourself to write; Schmidt & Alexander, 2012). The main point is that *emotions with writing are fluid and change over time.* In other words, graduate nursing students need to be prepared to feel different emotions at different times with different assignments. This is expected. Allowing space to experience whatever emotions surface will free most graduate nursing students from unnecessary self-judgment and self-criticism about where they should be and what they should be experiencing.

Once the self-judgment and self-criticism are minimized, most graduate nursing students can then move into a productive state of writing, even in the presence of emotions (i.e., fear, anxiety, dread). We provide concrete strategies later in this chapter to assist with moving into a productivity state.

As with any other situation involving an emotional response, give yourself time to process. For example, if you needed to reply to a colleague or peer via email regarding a conflicting topic, you would likely take a strategic pause before writing your response. You are giving yourself time to process and respond professionally. The strategic pause is common among authentic leaders and is extremely valuable during the writing and revision process.

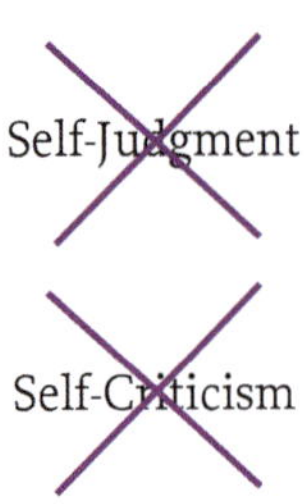

FIGURE 6.1 Silencing self-judgment and self-criticism.

Identifying the "I Should ..."

One of the most troubling obstacles to overcome while writing scholarly papers is the internal voice of "I should . . ." This internal dialogue can range from statements about what should be done to how one should be feeling. Generally, these comments are not positive, and if not quickly corrected can be damaging to motivation, productivity, and any joy in the writing process. These thoughts can also trigger unwanted emotional responses. Not only are the negative thoughts present, but so are the unsettling emotions, which can be challenging. One of the keys to preventing these hazardous emotions and thoughts is to listen to your internal dialogue. Once you "catch" the thoughts, you can more easily change your mind-set, leading toward a more positive and enjoyable writing experience. See Table 6.1 for sample "I should" statements and how you can reframe your thoughts.

TABLE 6.1 Identifying and Reframing Statements

Statements	Feedback	Reframed Statements
I am going too slow. This should not take so long.	*Writing can be an excruciatingly slow process. This is normal. Try not to judge your progress (or lack thereof).*	Yes, I am writing slower than previously. But I'm still writing.
I should be able to write more clearly; I know my clinical problem very well.	*Maybe your writing is not clear, but maybe your clinical problem is not that easy to understand. Writing brings clarity. You will get there.*	I am glad I recognize my writing lacks clarity. I will revisit and see how I can explain this better.
I should be motivated to write this paper; it's my last one of the semester!	*Maintaining motivation for a paper at the end of the semester is difficult. You are probably tired. This is all right.*	I can set aside some time for writing to take the stress off my plate. My motivation is the end of the semester.
I should be better at grammar. I've been writing my whole life.	*Grammar does not come naturally for everyone. It is like any other skill, and you refine as you learn.*	I have more to learn to master my grammar. I have made great strides so far.
I should not be so anxious about this small assignment.	*Anxiety can strike anywhere and at any time.*	It's OK to be anxious about any assignment. I will start writing when I am ready.

Cultural Dialogue Surrounding Writing

Our culture romanticizes the writing process. Ideas such as "waiting for inspiration to strike" or "generating words in extreme moments of productivity" are some examples of the unrealistic expectations for writing. Some of these concepts can be challenging to overcome because the ideas exist outside of academia. Graduate nursing students may hear these concepts in their personal or professional lives and start to believe some of the dialogue. As a result, these stereotypical perspectives can negatively impact students' attitudes and beliefs surrounding writing and can lead to challenging emotional responses (see Table 6.2).

Our goal is for you to become aware of phenomena external to academia. Listen to the dialogue around you. If the dialogue leads to more "I should" thinking and negative emotional responses, we encourage you to stop the thought and reframe. This constant back and forth is sometimes necessary for students (and faculty) who may struggle with various pieces within the writing process.

TABLE 6.2 Bringing Reality to Writing

False Cultural Commentary About Writing	Reality
Writers want to write.	*Maybe. Depends on the day. This cannot be said for all.*
Writers are often inspired and have the discipline for their craft.	*Maybe. Not always the case. Most writers struggle to find inspiration and struggle even more with the discipline needed to write.*
Writers have a natural draw to writing, and writing is not difficult for them.	*Yes, some writers may be naturally inclined to write, but this does not mean the craft is "easy." Much goes on beneath the surface.*
Scholarly writing is not as fun as fictional, creative writing.	*This could be true. But let's hope that we can all find some fun in scholarly writing!*

Fear

One of the most common emotions surrounding writing is fear. This may appear as fear of failure, fear of rejection, fear of not being good enough, fear of criticism, or fear of success. The list is endless, but the underlying emotion is fear. Often graduate nursing students have difficulty naming the type of fear, which can present in a variety of numerous behaviors such as procrastination, perfectionism, paralysis, rushing, or dissociating. Refer to the self-inventory described in Chapter 1 to best identify how fear presents for you.

Some of our most impactful (negative) emotions around writing stem from a challenging experience. If you hold some more negative memories that may warrant additional mental health guidance, we encourage you to work through the emotions with a trusted professional. Regardless of your level of comfort with any challenging emotions, we encourage you to be gentle with yourself in the writing experience. Watch your thoughts and attitudes surrounding writing and revise, if needed. Lastly, it is also important to note that it is possible to replace feelings from previous negative experiences with future positive experiences. Identifying a willing positive mentor or peer may be beneficial during a specific writing journey to replace negative writing experiences with positive ones.

Lack of Interest

Aside from any traumatic experiences with writing, many nursing graduate students express a lack of interest in writing (and reading) for pleasure. The environment of graduate school can be very demanding, with frequent reading and writing assignments, which can ultimately rid many students of the desire to read or write for pleasure. Writing for scholarly assignments can be even more difficult if graduate nursing students have no joy in the actual act of writing. To remedy this, we recommend ways to generate interest in what you write (and read). Adult learners are more likely to thrive in situations relevant to practice-focused knowledge and intrinsic and extrinsic motivational factors. See Table 6.3 for suggestions to enhance your writing and learning enjoyment.

Our suggestions are rooted in the idea that if students enjoy what they are learning (or enjoy some facet of the material), they will have a pleasurable experience, thereby reinforcing the content. That is our hope for you: to have fun with writing!

TABLE 6.3 Ways to Generate Interest in Writing

Ways to Generate Interest	Examples
Get curious	▪ Allow yourself to be curious. Use your assignment as a way to learn about something you've always been interested in. ▪ Allow yourself to ask questions. Write these questions down. Keep a running list.
Write about something that is specific to your interest* **Most graduate school assignments allow students to pick their topics.*	▪ Write about what you are interested in clinically. ▪ Draw on your experiences at the bedside and in your personal world.
Make time to read "fun" articles	▪ Read your favorite social media page. ▪ Set aside time to read magazine articles of niche interests (fashion, music, entertainment). ▪ Indulge in guilty pleasure reading. ▪ Set aside personal time for reading to bring joy.

Clinical Practice and Former Coursework

Scholarly writing may not align with the daily tasks of clinical practice. As a result, many graduate nursing students find motivation challenging and fleeting. Additionally, students may question the usefulness of these skills outside of the classroom. All of these reasons can lead to negative emotional responses, which in turn can make writing more difficult. See Table 6.4, which outlines the process of reframing perspectives rooted in clinical experiences.

We encourage you to sit with the emotions as they arise. In fact, you may experience the emotion before identifying the thought. This is normal and to be expected. Use the emotion as a signal that you may need to trace back to the thought. You can then move forward with reframing the thoughts and settling into a more positive outlook.

TABLE 6.4 Reframing Clinical Perspectives

Clinical Perspectives →	Possible Emotions →	Reframed Thoughts
I'll never use these skills in the hospital.	▪ Frustration ▪ Doubt ▪ Anger	▪ This will help me be succinct and convincing.
These writing assignments have nothing to do with my job.	▪ Irritation ▪ Apprehension ▪ Distress	▪ I will be a well-rounded nurse and have the skills to excel at any level.
I just want to learn how to write good notes, not academic papers.	▪ Contempt ▪ Bitterness ▪ Hostility	▪ The skills are transferrable; I will do well at both.

Imposter Syndrome

Single emotions such as fear or anxiety can manifest into larger, more robust concepts. One of the most frequently discussed (and researched) topics surrounding academic performance is imposter syndrome. This is not particularly a "syndrome" in the clinical sense but does have significant features and manifestations, which can present for many graduate nursing students (and even faculty). Imposter syndrome is a complex set of interrelated emotions (fear, self-doubt, disbelief) in which a person feels like a fraud within their profession or discipline and will eventually be caught. These complex emotions usually stem from a variety of reasons related to situations, personality, and behavioral traits.

Clance and Imes (1978) first identified this phenomenon after studying self-perception among 150 high-achieving (i.e., successful in their respective careers) women in the United States. The authors of this groundbreaking study revealed that their participants felt they were unworthy of praise and success despite providing participants with evidence of their value (Clance & Imes, 1978). In other words, the participants were unable to acknowledge their worthiness of praise and success.

Imposter syndrome is prevalent in a variety of work settings, but most frequently appears in academia. Graduate nursing students may feel pressure to perform and achieve success through making high grades (even though the ultimate tests of accomplishment are with the licensing boards). Nursing faculty members also struggle with imposter syndrome due to the pressure to publish high-quality papers, maintain optimism within peer review processes, and compete nationally for research grants. While the concept of imposter syndrome appears across multiple disciplines and professions, several studies suggest that the rates are higher among nursing students, nurse practitioners, and nurse scientists (Gill, 2020; Parkman, 2016).

If you suspect you may experience imposter syndrome, please refer to the following quiz from Valerie Young (2011):

1. Do you chalk your success up to luck, timing, or computer error?
2. Do you believe "If I can do it, anybody can"?
3. Do you agonize over the smallest flaws in your work?
4. Are you crushed by even constructive criticism, seeing it as evidence of your ineptness?
5. When you do succeed, do you secretly feel you fooled them again?
6. Do you worry that it's just a matter of time before you're "found out"?

For an alternate version (2022) of this quiz, see https://impostorsyndrome.com/infographics/impostor-syndrome-quiz/.

Graduate nursing students who identify with imposter syndrome will have to pay particular attention to their internal thoughts. This is mostly achieved through self-reflection and fostering of an attitude of lifelong learning. Additionally, learning to receive and manage critical peer feedback will help reduce the pressure of perfect performance associated with imposter syndrome. (Additional information about peer feedback is covered in Chapter 9.) Furthermore, graduate nursing students and faculty often overestimate the success others (peers and colleagues) and underestimate the energy, struggles, and time needed to reach certain goals (Gill, 2020). Adding awareness about the unseen efforts and failures of others may help reduce any burden or pressure accompanying imposter syndrome. Lastly, working with effective mentors and engaging with safe peers can serve as a positive experience to help combat the doubt associated with imposter syndrome. While imposter syndrome is likely to never to fully subside, you can slowly build confidence with time and reminders of success.

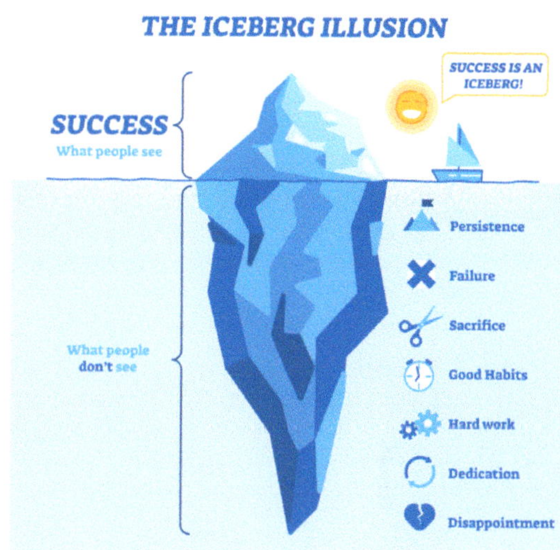

FIGURE 6.2 The iceberg illusion of success.

One of our own writers of this book shares her experiences with imposter syndrome:

> No matter how many articles I have published or grants I have successfully funded, I often stress and worry about the quality of my work and if I'm "doing enough." Historically, I have attributed these feelings to neuroticism. However, they really stem farther back to imposter syndrome—which, for me, is the idea that one day someone very important is going to rescind all my research and work, and the thought that someday I will be "caught"—that I really don't know what I am doing, and all of my

work has been phony. As outlandish as this may seem, literature suggests that up to 70% of people have experienced some form of imposter syndrome at some point of their lives. However, there is some good news if you suffer from imposter syndrome. Techniques such as reflection, lifelong learning attitudes, and peer support can be effective in combating imposter syndrome.

Albert Einstein said it best, "The difference between what the most and the least learned people know is inexpressibly trivial in relation to that which is unknown."
– Elizabeth Riley, DNP, APRN, CPNP-AC, PED-BC, RNC-NIC, CNE, ANEF

References

Clance, P. R., & Imes, S. (1978). The imposter phenomenon in high achieving women: Dynamics and therapeutic intervention. *Psychotherapy Theory, Research and Practice, 15*(3), 241–247.

Gill, P. (2020). Imposter syndrome: Why is it so common among nurse researchers and is it really a problem? *Nurse Researcher, 28*(3), 30–36.

Parkman, A. (2016). The imposter phenomenon in higher education: Incidence and impact. *Journal of Higher Education Theory and Practice, 16*(1), 51–60.

Schmidt, K. M., & Alexander, J. E. (2012). The empirical development of an instrument to measure writerly self-efficacy in writing centers. *The Journal of Writing Assessment, 5*(1), 1–10. http://www.journalofwritingassessment.org/article.php?article=62

Young, V. (2011). *The secret thoughts of successful women: Why capable people suffer from the imposter syndrome and how to thrive in spite of it.* Penguin.

Credit

CHAPTER 7

The Thing No One Likes to Talk About

Discipline to Write

Pearman D. Parker and Elizabeth Riley

The prior chapter was about emotions surrounding writing. Graduate nursing students and most writers learn to navigate through, with, and around the emotions. Here we will talk about a necessary skill needed to write: discipline.

What Is Discipline?

Merriam-Webster (2022b) defines *discipline* as "control gained by enforcing obedience or order; orderly or prescribed conduct or pattern of behavior." Some associations for this word may include order, control, and patterns. The same can be applied to writing.

We define disciplined writing as the repetitive application of time and energy into a writing project. As we have previously mentioned (see Chapter 1), scholarly writing includes more than just generating words. Discipline is required for all elements of writing. Examples include scheduling dates/times each week on your calendar to write or blocking out 1 hour in your weekly schedule just for thinking time (reading journal articles, asking questions, brainstorming outlines). Before we delve too far into the specific skills needed to write with discipline, let's process with the following self-inventory:

Take a moment to check-in with yourself.

- What does the word *discipline* mean to you?
- What feelings, thoughts, or attitudes come up for you?
- Are these positive or negative?
- How else can you reframe your feelings, thoughts, or attitudes about discipline for writing?

Here are some suggestions for reframing your thoughts:

Initial Thoughts on Writing and Discipline	**Reframing the Thought**
Discipline makes writing sound hard. I'm already struggling to get started.	Discipline is just showing up even when I don't feel like it. If I contribute some time to this project, eventually I will start.
Discipline sounds like more for me to do. I am already at my max. I can't add on any more stress right now.	I'm overwhelmed and that's OK. I will carve out 15 minutes tomorrow morning to think about my project. It will help my anxiety in the long term.
This seems so unnecessary for my clinical work. I don't need to write every day.	No, I don't need to write every day, but I want to reduce my stress on the front end, so I'll go ahead and get started to help myself in the future.

What Are the Components of Disciplined Writing?

We previously defined disciplined writing as the "repetitive application of time and energy into a writing project." This abstract definition is broad and applicable to various writers and nursing students. However, this definition does not identify the specific characteristics needed to create, maintain, and sustain a working writing discipline. These characteristics are as follows: time, resiliency, commitment, and receptiveness.

Time

Merriam-Webster (2022e) defines *time* as the "the measured or measurable period during which an action, process, or condition exists or continues." Yet, time is simultaneously one of the most complex concepts within the discipline of writing. The element of time is a mysterious, dynamic concept and is something most nursing students should strive to master. Whether you are trying to meet deadlines or planning in advance for your writing, time is highly valuable. We encourage you to think about your own history of working with (or against) time with the following self-inventory questions:

Take a moment to check in with yourself.

- What is your relationship with time and writing?
- What are your patterns when working under deadlines?
- Do you usually meet the deadlines far in advance or work until the last minute? Maybe you have a sweet spot of planning ahead and working a little every day?
- What are some factors that have unexpectedly derailed your use of time?
- Think about your own personal projects outside of writing that require an element of using time (i.e., planning parties, weddings, vacations). What was that experience like? Did you enjoy the process? How similar or different was planning that event(s) to writing?

The self-inventory about your relationship with time may have been revealing or illuminated very little. Many professional writers have a complex relationship with time and develop personal strategies to manage their time. Similarly, many nursing students and nursing faculty constantly are faced with issues surrounding time. For example, graduate nursing students may have unexpected course assignments or unplanned life events that derail their planning. Nursing faculty may have to delay writing time to meet greater priorities of work commitments. The overarching point here is that time impacts everyone, including graduate nursing students.

We recommend that graduate nursing students use time as a protective structure. Set writing times on a daily, weekly, or biweekly basis can help students become more accountable and productive. The structure of using set times can relieve graduate nursing students of the pressure of trying to "find" creativity or "wait for the inspiration," which is prevalent in much of today's cultural discussion surrounding writing. Instead, we want to encourage you to use time in a structured manner to help you meet your goals and deadlines. For example, daily writing time of 30 minutes or less can significantly reduce anxiety and, consequently, procrastination. Additionally, having a dedicated writing time can allow graduate nursing students to fill their time with other priorities while knowing that their writing time is already scheduled for the week. The amount of time required to perfect disciplined writing can vary for each person, but here are some suggestions that may be helpful in your discipline development.

As you read through these suggestions, please remember that each item may or may not work. You may have to revisit some of these approaches depending on your needs and the environment of your life at the time. Some of these suggestions are adapted from a faculty-centered scholarly writing resource of "The Writer's Block," "Write & Recharge," and the "Immersive Writing Retreat" (Franks, 2018).

- Block out minutes to hours of your daily schedule to just write. Minimize distractions (close email, close all nonwriting windows, etc.) during this time.
- Maintain consistent times for your writing. This will help define a habit.
- Be aware of how you use time. Check the clocks, set timers, and so forth. This will give you additional structure and reduce the chance of burnout.
- Protect your blocked time. Do not allow for additional meetings during this time. Treat your writing time as a meeting.
- Celebrate when you meet your writing goals.
- Give yourself grace even if you do not meet your goals within the time frame.
- Allow yourself to make errors during the writing process (i.e., not protecting your time, getting caught up in emails, watching a new television show while trying to write, etc.).
- Assume that you will need more time.
- Give yourself more time at the beginning to allow for unexpected stressors (in professional and personal life).
- Follow your time schedules. Reward yourself by stopping at the designated time. This will help you avoid burnout.

Resiliency

Resiliency is fundamental to maintaining a writing discipline. Merriam-Webster (2022d) defines *resiliency* as "an ability to recover from or adjust easily to adversity or change." Disciplined writing is similar to the dedication required for perfecting any hobby or sport. As you train in a sport, you will experience hardships and setbacks, but ideally, you do not stop with your training. The same goes for writing: You will experience hardships, frustrations, and setbacks but maintaining the discipline (e.g., practice) of writing is key to success.

We previously discussed the emotional hardships associated with writing (see Chapter 6). The emotional responses can be draining for many people and can be especially difficult for graduate nursing students who are already juggling multiple class assignments, clinical placements, and personal life situations. If not monitored and corrected for, burnout is a natural consequence. Burnout is the result of prolonged stress. Symptoms include exhaustion, feelings of cynicism, and detachment from work or course studies (Maslach & Leiter, 2016). Resiliency is the key to preventing burnout and is something that develops over time with intention and with many experiences (Wei et al., 2019). Please take the time to reflect on your experiences with burnout toward writing with the following self-inventory:

Symptoms of burnout in writing:

- being exhausted and unable to generate ideas, thoughts, or words
- hopelessness toward writing
- feelings of depletion and depressive symptoms surrounding writing
- experiences with writing affecting personal and professional life

Note: Please seek outside, emotionally safe support if you experience these symptoms before returning to tackle your writing projects. Sometimes support and rest are the best medicine. Your discipline with writing is part of what you do, not who you are.

We recommend that graduate nursing students make efforts to promote resiliency prior to experiencing burnout. Some of the strategies are simple cognitive reframing, and others are approaches we found useful with our own writing. Please stay aware of your own emotional and mental health needs. Your wellness is a priority over any discipline.

Take a moment to reflect on these strategies. You may already be using these strategies in your professional and personal life. Please continue what works for you and try other strategies when you feel ready.

1. Reframe negative, self-defeating thoughts.
   a. I'll never get this. I've revised it so many times. It will never be good enough. I am not a good writer. → My revisions are making my paper better. I got this. I am learning.
2. Remember your dedication to your scholarly product.
   a. Think back to the time when you first came up with your idea for your writing product. Remember that enthusiasm. That energy did not go anywhere; invite the excitement back into your work.
3. Tend to your physical needs.
   a. Make sure you are writing with your best self—your best attitude, mind-set, presence (if, and when, possible).
   b. Writing can be mentally exhausting and tiring. Make sure you are getting enough quality sleep.
   c. Manage your diet best for your body.
   d. Get exercise. If writing during large time periods, be sure to set your timer and move every 45 minutes or hour. If necessary, set your timer and reward your writing time with walks, meditation, exercise, or anything that you enjoy.
4. Allow for time to develop resiliency.
   a. Resiliency with writing develops over time, as with any sport, hobby, or skill. Give yourself grace as you develop the resiliency muscle for the writing discipline.

Commitment

A concept similar to resiliency is commitment. Developing a strong discipline to writing takes a level of commitment to the act of writing, to your scholarly product, and to improving your skills. Merriam-Webster (2022a) defines *commitment* as "an agreement or pledge to do something in the future." We define commitment to writing as the internal agreement to continue writing despite significant stressors. When challenges arise or burnout occurs, remembering the commitment to your writing can provide fuel to seek support, rest, and, ultimately, continue. We encourage you to think about your own history of commitment with the following self-inventory questions:

Take a moment to reflect on these thoughts.

1. Reflect on a few experiences in which you wanted to quit but persevered because you were dedicated to a goal. What ultimately kept you going?

2. Think about your commitment to writing. How can you apply those same experiences with commitment to your writing?

3. How might you increase or maintain your level of commitment to writing?

4. What goals do you have with your own scholarly writing?

5. Brainstorm some ways to maintain your commitment.

Most graduate nursing students believe commitment to writing has an end point, which is usually the end of a course or program. In other words, their commitment to writing only extends to a relatively short time period. One beneficial change of thought may be to maintain a commitment to writing for a lifetime. While this may seem a bit overwhelming and unnecessary, taking a longer view of developing skills over a lifetime relieves the immediate pressure of having to learn and refine all the writing skills in a short period of time. Additionally, maintaining a longer commitment to writing beyond a class or year can help graduate nursing students retain newly acquired writing knowledge and apply the writing skills we discuss in this book.

Review these strategies initially as you would with a hobby or sport. Then read them again with writing in mind. If you feel any anxiety or emotional unrest, move your mind back to your hobby or sport (ideally something you enjoy). Keep doing this until your confidence increases with your own level of commitment to writing. Please note your commitment may wax or wane depending on life and environmental circumstances. This is normal. Giving yourself grace within the disciplined writing is paramount.

1. Write down your reasons for wanting to be a better writer and place these reasons in a spot near your work (by a laptop, in your office, etc.). Whenever you feel the stressors of writing, refer to your reasons. They may serve as a reminder for your commitment.
2. Edit and revise your reasons when appropriate. Sometimes your reasons may change as you grow and develop. This is normal.
3. Give yourself grace. You will not always maintain a particular level of commitment to the discipline of writing. Do not criticize yourself. Simply remind yourself of your dedication or reasons and start again (when ready).
4. Use every writing task as an opportunity to practice good, effective writing. This includes texts, emails, letters, and even messages on social media. Adding more awareness to your writing outside of the classroom will help you stay committed to the discipline of writing.

Receptiveness

The last component needed to cultivate a discipline of writing is being willing to improve your work, skills, and knowledge. This willingness to consider, to accept, or to improve based on new suggestions or ideas is referred to as receptiveness. Merriam-Webster (2022c) defines *receptiveness* as "open and responsive to ideas, impressions." We define receptiveness in writing as the willingness to adjust. Maintaining receptiveness when writing is essential. Some graduate nursing students close off (or reject) feedback once they start making high marks on their papers. Other students may believe they have mastered writing and do not need to spend any more time improving their skills since they already do well on their assignments. In both of these scenarios the result is a lack of growth. As mentioned earlier, maintaining a lifelong commitment to writing will help you be open, as writing is one skill that can always be improved.

Examples of receptiveness:

1. Think about feedback and then respond; do not immediately dismiss.
2. Explore other ways to improve grammar and content (e.g., meeting with a tutor, reading peers' work, exposing yourself to other quality writers).
3. Try new approaches to time management (e.g., setting timers or rewarding with breaks) or stress reduction (e.g., mindful body movement, meditation, dance, etc.) when needed.
4. Talk to your friends about your struggles with writing. Ask them how they handled or dealt with particular situations.

5. Read books, blogs, social media pages, or websites about ways to improve your writing.
6. Identify and read quality written work among nurses and other disciplines. Think about what elements you liked and how you can incorporate such into your own work.
7. Welcome learning about writing techniques, strategies, approaches, and skills. Remember, this is a lifelong practice!

Remaining open to change and adjustment to writing concepts and skills can be challenging, especially during frustrating or stressful events (e.g., receiving unsolicited feedback on a particularly difficult manuscript draft). We cover ways to receive such feedback (see Chapter 9), but openness is fundamental.

Application of Disciplined Writing

The core elements of disciplined writing include time, resiliency, commitment, and receptiveness. Graduate nursing students must understand each of these concepts and apply such skills to create, manage, and maintain a discipline to writing. See Table 7.1 for examples of applying these skills.

TABLE 7.1 Concepts and Examples

Concept	Skills	Application to Nursing Students
Time	Dedicate daily writing time.	Write every Tuesday and Thursday from 9:00–10:00 a.m.
	Commit to your writing time.	Allow writing breaks during holidays or vacations.
	Maintain awareness of time.	
	Be protective of this time.	Set deadlines with peers; ask for weekly progress check-ins.
Resiliency	Catch negative thoughts and reframe.	"I'll never get this → I am getting this."
	Allow for breaks.	Take a 10-minute break for every 50 minutes of writing.
	Give yourself grace, as you are always learning.	"This is really hard, but I believe in my purpose as a nurse."
	Remember enthusiasm .	"I am stressed about this assignment, but I am on my way to graduating!"

Commitment	Set visual reminders of your commitment to writing. Revise and/or add more writing goals when appropriate. Give yourself grace when needed.	Place Post-It notes of writing goals you want to achieve on your laptop. Celebrate when you meet a writing goal (can be as small as writing a paragraph or large such as getting a manuscript accepted). Resting after a major setback and then picking back up again when ready.
Receptiveness	Allow for new suggestions to improve your writing. Seek expert help when doubting. Welcome new changes to your writing skills.	Talk about your struggles with published authors or nursing faculty. Ask them how they work around or with obstacles. Read various writing books and find one(s) that resonate with you the most. Try working with professional editors or join writing communities online.

References

Franks, A. M. (2018). Design and evaluation of a longitudinal faculty development program to advance scholarly writing among pharmacy practice faculty. *American Journal of Pharmaceutical Education, 82*(6), 654–659. https://doi.org/10.5688/ajpe6556

Maslach, C., & Leiter, M. P. (2016). Understanding the burnout experience: Recent research and its implications for psychiatry. *World Psychiatry, 15*(2), 103–111. https://doi.org/10.1002/wps.20311

Merriam-Webster. (2022a). *Commitment.* https://www.merriam-webster.com/dictionary/commitment

Merriam-Webster. (2022b). *Discipline.* https://www.merriam-webster.com/dictionary/discipline

Merriam-Webster. (2022c). *Openness.* https://www.merriam-webster.com/dictionary/openness

Merriam-Webster. (2022d). *Resiliency.* https://www.merriam-webster.com/dictionary/resiliency

Merriam-Webster. (2022e). *Time.* https://www.merriam-webster.com/dictionary/time

Wei, H., Roberts, P., Strickler, J., & Corbett, R. W. (2019). Nurse leaders' strategies to foster nurse resilience. *Journal of Nursing Management, 27*(4), 681–687. https://doi.org/10.1111/jonm.12736

CHAPTER 8

Conducting, Receiving, and Responding to Peer Review

Samuel R. Atcherson and Pearman D. Parker

> *I love science. I hate supposition, superstition, exaggeration and falsified data. Show me the research, show me the results, show me the conclusions—and then show me some qualified peer reviews of all that.*
>
> —Bill Vaughan

Peer review has been around since the beginning of humankind; however, its formal use is believed to have begun when philosophical and scientific information was shared widely with the development and improvement of the printing press, such as Johannes Gutenberg's press. As a consequence, duplicates of written work could be made and shared broadly. The printing press is credited for increasing literacy and education in Europe. With increased literacy and education, however, came opportunities for feedback, scrutiny, skepticism, and debate.

The *Philosophical Transactions of the Royal Society* is thought to be the first journal to formalize the peer review process in the mid-1660s, when founding editor, Henry Oldenburg, submitted essays for review to individuals he considered subject matter experts. The underlying purpose of this activity was the concern that accuracy and truthfulness of written works could not be guaranteed unless they were reviewed by other expert peers. Indeed, the peer review practice continues to this day in many areas and is considered a hallmark feature for most academic and scientific writing. The rigor of peer review adds an additional layer of confidence in the validity of the scholarly product. While the peer review system has received extensive criticism in recent years (Haffar et al., 2019), we believe in the inherit value of presenting work to a small group of expert peers as one last final check before disseminating the work to a larger, international community of scientists and to the public.

Purpose of Peer Review

The Merriam-Webster (2022) dictionary defines *peer review* as "a process by which something proposed (as for research or publication) is evaluated by a group of experts in the appropriate field." In practice, a peer review is any process by which a peer can evaluate and provide feedback to another peer. Generally, rank within a group (e.g., undergraduate class, level of professor) is not taken into consideration. Instead, you and your peers are grouped into broad categories (e.g., students, faculty, leaders; see Table 8.1).

TABLE 8.1 Examples of Peers Conducting Peer Review

Type of Peer Group	Members of Peer Group	Materials Reviewed
Nursing students	▪ Undergraduate students (junior, senior) ▪ Graduate students (PhD, MSN, DNP)	▪ Class assignments ▪ Clinical care plans ▪ Assessment notes ▪ Class papers and presentations
Nursing faculty and clinical instructors	▪ Assistant, associate, and full professors ▪ Clinical instructors	▪ Syllabi ▪ Course materials ▪ Teaching observations ▪ Clinical evaluations ▪ Clinical skills ▪ Promotion and tenure materials
Nursing leaders	▪ Chief nursing officers, chief executive officers ▪ Hospital administrators ▪ Nurse directors, managers	▪ Handbooks ▪ Policies and procedures ▪ Strategic plans ▪ Budgets ▪ Accreditation materials
Nurse scientists	▪ PhD-prepared nursing faculty engaging in research in academia, public/private organizations	▪ Grant applications ▪ Manuscripts ▪ Podium and poster abstracts ▪ Presentations ▪ Book chapters

As the focus of this book is on writing, the remainder of this chapter will focus on the peer review process for written materials.

Types of Peer Review

There are multiple types of peer review for written materials that graduate nursing students might encounter in their educational training and career (Author Hub, n.d.):

- Single-blind peer review
    - This type of peer review occurs when the authors are blind to whom the reviewers are. This protects the individual reviewers, but because the reviewers know who the author is, their decision may be shaped by their views on any of the authors' other works, which may be biased.
- Double-blind peer review
    - This type of peer review occurs when the identity of both authors and reviewers are blind to each other. Specifically, this would require all names and affiliations to be removed (usually in the title page and any attributions to hospitals/institutions made in the manuscript), and thus protects both the authors and reviewers.
- Open peer review
    - This type of peer review occurs when the authors and reviewers are known to each other. Generally, the reviewers provide comments and will openly sign that the comments came from them.
- Collaborative peer review
    - This type of peer review often involves more than one reviewer who offer comments in a joint fashion (i.e., Reviewer 1, Reviewer 2) and may confer with both the author and editor during the review process. This is one of the most common peer-review methods.
- Third-party peer review
    - This type of peer review involves an independent review service before an author submits somewhere officially. This approach may be helpful for manuscripts requiring content and language editing.
- Post-publication peer review
    - This type of peer review is one that occurs after publication is complete, but an open forum opportunity is created to permit further comments and discussion about the publication. Here, the original reviewers may also have their names and comments published, along with the publication.

- Cascading peer review
  - This type of peer review is one that can occur if a submission was previously reviewed, but the outcome did not result in acceptance. There are many reasons a submission may not be accepted. However, in cascading peer review, the authors may use the results of any prior review to revise, improve, or build on that work for submission elsewhere.

How to Conduct a Peer Review

In the previous section, we described numerous types of peer review. Regardless of the type of peer review, we there are some basic steps to conduct a peer review:

- Understand the expectations.
  - It helps peer reviewers when they understand how the written work is to be evaluated. This can be provided in the form of written expectations, such as a set of criteria or rubric. Written expectations, criteria, and rubrics can help give the review some structure. Some peer reviews can be more informal and subjective, whereas others are formal and a bit more objective. Once you understand how the written work is to be evaluated, your brain will be primed to look for certain things in your review.
- Get your materials ready.
  - If the review will be paper based, it helps to have a pencil or pen ready. If the review will take place electronically or digitally, such as on a computer or portable tablet, consider what is acceptable for when you conduct your thorough read and takes notes. Regardless of the method used, be sure to have a preplanned method for completing and submitting feedback for the review.
- Scan the work for organization.
  - Before you start your thorough read and start taking notes, get a quick sense for how the written product is organized. Read the title, abstract, and conclusions or summary to prime yourself for the review, and take then a moment to identify keywords, headings, subheadings, references, and any tables, figures, or supplements. For a journal article, book, or book chapter, it helps to read the published "Instructions for Authors." For grant applications, it helps to read through the guidelines provided in the call for applications. For other types of written materials, such course assignments, it helps to consult with the instructor, and/or the syllabus, and/or the rubrics for the assignment.

- Conduct a thorough read and take notes.
    - Now that you know what is expected, have your materials ready, and have an overview of the written work, it is time to carve out some time to conduct a thorough read and start taking notes in the margins. Conversely, a reviewer can use a numbering system whereby a number is written next to the item in question, and on a separate document makes notes in numbered order. Regardless of which method is used, the reviewer will have information helpful to the author to use for improvement and/or revision. As you work on this step, it may be helpful to ask yourself questions such as these:

Sample peer review questions to guide feedback:

- Does the article show the "the big picture"?
- Does the title match the content of the paper?
- Does the paper have logical flow?
- Are abbreviations used and spelled out appropriately in the right order?
- Do the authors make the case for the purpose of the written work, including any research questions asked?
- Are ideas presented clearly?
- Is the writing clear and free from major spelling and grammatical mistakes?
- If there are methods, are the methods clear and replicable?
- If data was collected, is the data presented in a meaningful way, and do the statistical procedures appear to be appropriate?
- Are there any inconsistencies or errors?
- Are the references appropriate or relevant?
- Is any thing missing or irrelevant?
- Do the authors present any strengths or limitations?

- Complete the review.
    - Offer results of your evaluation

Completion of the review takes place when the thorough reading and note taking are finished. Depending on the expectations for the peer review, the reviewers now have the opportunity to summarize their understanding of the written work and/or offer point-by-point feedback.

- Reconcile the introduction and conclusions.

In your mind, are you able to reconcile the introduction with the conclusions? In other words, does the introduction make the case or set the tone for the entire written work? Does the conclusion effectively wrap things up to include connecting all the subpoints with the major points? If not, be sure to provide feedback to the authors.

- Offer questions and suggestions.

Authors generally appreciate feedback, particularly when it is positive or provides suggestions for improvement. Peer reviewers can offer precise and exact suggestions to fix issues, but they can also ask questions as suggestions for improvement.

Sample feedback from a peer reviewer:

- The title of your paper does not seem to match the content well. Could a revised title be more effective?
- You use multiple terms through the paper for the same concept, but it makes reading very difficult. Can you pick a term and use that consistently?
- This section seems out of place and abrupt. Is there better place in the paper to move this?
- This sentence appears to be a run-on and unclear. Can you resolve this so that it is easier to understand?
- Would this information be better presented in a table format?

Above all, peer reviewers should offer their feedback in a kind and respectful manner. However, this is not always the case. Some reviewers can be rude and unhelpful in their critique of the writing. This can be devastating for not only nursing students but seasoned, expert faculty as well. We will discuss some strategies in the section "How to Receive Peer Review" when dealing with a variety of feedback—both encouraging and disappointing.

Examples of Recommendations for Manuscript Peer Review

Peer reviewers generally offer editors three main suggestions before articles (manuscripts) are accepted for publication:

- Accept with minor revisions: The manuscript is generally of sound methods, argument development, and meets the rigorous criteria for publication of the particular journal. Minor revisions such as copy editing (word choices, sentence structure) can be expected.

- Revise and resubmit: The manuscript may need additional work before being fully accepted for publication. Revisions may include adding content, expanding on an argument, further describing methods, or explaining study design rationale. Additionally, revisions may be requested multiple times depending on the level of work needed for the manuscript and reviewers' preferences.

- Reject: The manuscript is not suitable for publication of the particular journal. Reasons may or may not be explained.

How to Receive Peer Review

Chances are you will be subject to peer review of your own work at some point in your educational training or career. Receiving a review from your peers can be quite uncomfortable, especially since you have likely invested a great deal of time and energy in your written work. When it comes to work that will make its way into the public domain (especially the scientific community), we should want our work to have meaning and usefulness and be high quality so that we are neither wasting our time nor theirs.

When you receive the review of your work, take a moment to ground yourself; take a few deeps breaths, and get into the right mind-set to be open to the comments and feedback. Be prepared for a reviewer's objectivity and subjectivity, along with their own humanity and lens through which they have experienced or encountered the topic you have written about. Nothing is to be taken personally; try to hone in to what your peer is trying to convey to you. Chances are, if something does not make sense to them, it may also may not make sense to others.

In the event you receive harsh criticism that may be unkind or even cruel, we advise you to seek support from emotionally safe peers and/or mentors. Receiving feedback, especially when sharp, can be especially damaging to one's confidence. Your peers and mentors can be an invaluable source of support as you navigate through the responses. While some feedback may be worthy of consideration, we recommend that you ensure your emotional health with support before tackling the feedback and responding or submitting to a new journal.

How to Respond to Peer Review

In the event that you have the opportunity to revise and resubmit your written work to the same (or different) peer reviewers, it can really help to organize reviewer comments and your responses in a table format. An example of response to internal peer review feedback is provided in Table 8.2 for a recently accepted manuscript submitted to the *Journal of Psychosocial Nursing and Mental Health Services* on a phenomenological study of deaf lipreaders during universal masking as a result of the COVID-19 pandemic (Carroll & Atcherson, in press). Here, the authors carefully read each reviewer comment and responded back to them individually. Where appropriate, they indicated what changes they made to the original manuscript. To reduce the burden during the second (or more) reviews, track changes or highlights may be applied by the authors to make it easier for the reviewers to judge whether changes have been made at a reasonable or satisfactory level. There may be times when you disagree with the reviewers, and you can offer a respectful rebuttal to back up your argument when appropriate.

TABLE 8.2 Example Responses by Authors to Peer Reviewer

Peer Reviewer Comment	Response From Authors
Although this might be outside of a traditional interpretive phenomenological study, some of the quotes seem to indicate tremendous sadness and anger. Did any of the participants ask for a referral for help? If so, how did you handle that? I think of your question "What was it like for you as a lipreader during this time of COVID when society is masked?" as similar to asking our patients questions related to depression or pain. If we ask those types of questions, and an individual responds positively, we need to do something about that. For example, how did you handle the response "I've had many breakdowns and cried myself to sleep because I cannot 'hear' in today's world."	The goal of this study was to phenomenologically capture the experience. Many respondents spoke of the experience negatively but then spoke of how they learned to cope with the experience over time. No participants asked for a referral for help. We did not feel any referrals were warranted based on how the interviews progressed and how the participants expressed their coping strategies and solutions. ▪ *Please see the polite response from the authors in which they acknowledged the reviewer but were able to defend their choices for the referrals.*
As noted on page 6, "Thematic Analysis occurred concurrently with data collection, Thematic techniques of Benner (1994) were used, . . ." What are the stages/phases of Benner's techniques? How were these phases used in this study?	As we used the commonalities seen in Benner and Heidegger's approaches, we focused on the common elements of rereading the transcripts and focusing on contextual information. We used Benner's techniques to tease out the specific issues of embodiment, temporality, etc., and a sentence was added to clarify this approach. Our themes are related to these components, as these were used as a framework for our analysis. Under data analysis, we moved the sentence about Benner to integrate it in a clearer way within the overall data analysis. We also added a citation for Benner when describing exemplars to make it evident that this is part of Benner's approach. ▪ *Here is a good example of meeting the reviewer's questions. The authors moved the sentence for clarity and provided additional citations to add context.*
What are the authors' thoughts about the use of adaptive voice-enhancing technologies to minimize negative experiences of lipreaders in a masked society in the future?	Speech-to-text transcription has improved in accuracy over the past few years, but it still fails when there is background noise or when the person isn't speaking close enough to the microphone. This was addressed under practice implications and a clause about a quiet environment was added. ▪ *Here is a good example of the authors identifying where the revisions were made. This will help streamline the subsequent review.*

Conclusions

Peer review is a wonderful tool for the dissemination of information, especially in science, health care, and academia. Peer review can take place using a variety of different media and by a variety of different peers. The goal of peer review is to ensure not only accuracy and truthfulness, but also help promote high-quality and impactful information to a variety of audiences. Whether we receive or provide peer reviews, they should be approached with good intentions offering honest but constructive feedback, and with an open mind for improvement.

References

Author Hub. (n.d.). *A guide to peer reviewing journal articles.* Cambridge University Press. https://www.cambridge.org/core/services/aop-file-manager/file/5a1eb62e67f405260662a0df/Refreshed-Guide-Peer-Review-Journal.pdf

Carroll, S. M., & Atcherson, S. R. (in press). Living in a limited world: Experience of lipreaders when society is masked. *Journal of Psychosocial and Mental Health Nursing Services.*

Haffar, S., Bazerbachi, F., & Murad, M. H. (2019). Peer review bias: A critical review. *Mayo Clinic Proceedings, 94*(4), 670–676. https://doi.org/10.1016/j.mayocp.2018.09.004

Merriam-Webster. (2022). *Peer review.* https://www.merriam-webster.com/dictionary/peer%20review

CHAPTER 9

Responding to Criticism

How to Digest Feedback and Move Forward

Pearman D. Parker and Elizabeth Riley

Critique is a fundamental aspect to scholarly writing. Whether a writer gives a critique or receives critical feedback, the experience can be jarring. The result can be devastating for nursing students—so much so that many students lose significant amounts of confidence and belief in their work. While this is a common event, many writing books fail to acknowledge the possible shock associated with critique. We hope to provide you with real-world accounts of how a variety of scholars move beyond and navigate such criticisms. Though criticism never stops at a certain level, we believe that nursing students can learn skills now to handle such feedback. Before taking a self-inventory of your personal skills that help when receiving feedback, consider the variety of emotions and experiences of writers across disciplines. Our hope is that you find these stories humorous, relatable, and, above all, encouraging.

First Steps for Reading the Review

Receiving the peer review feedback for manuscripts, grant applications, or other scholarly written products can evoke much anxiety. Some writers have a variety of methods to best receive the information. Some tend to read the reviews all at once and then give themselves a few days before tackling the feedback. Other colleagues intentionally delay opening the review until they are in a good mind-set to receive the critique. Whatever you do to prepare yourself to receive feedback as a student, just make sure to go slowly at a pace best for your mental health and stress level. When in doubt, we encourage you to reach out to emotionally safe mentors and faculty members to help you process the feedback.

> When we receive peer review comments on a grant or manuscript, most of us tend to focus right away on the negative comments and criticisms. They seem to weigh heavier on us than the positive comments we may also receive. It is true that in writing a response to peer review comments, we have to mainly address the criticisms that were raised. However, upon receiving a peer review report, my advice is to be intentional about first acknowledging the strengths that are highlighted in the report. Those criticisms can wait a bit!
>
> —Marjan Boerma, PhD, Professor of Pharmaceutical Sciences

Framing Your Thoughts Around the Reviews

One of the best methods to process the reviews is to stay focused on the outcome: a stronger written scholarly product. The end goal is to publish your work that has been thoroughly reviewed and approved by peers and other experts. After you process the initial emotional responses, we encourage you to remember the end goal: Publish your manuscript or to receive a good grade on one of your class papers. Another point to take into consideration is that the reviews from peers or your faculty members are extremely time intensive. The work is unpaid and often time-consuming. Your peers and faculty members are donating their time and expertise to guide you to polish your final product. Sometimes this perspective is helpful when you work through the necessary revisions.

> Writing is a skill that develops over time with practice and error. Your success depends on your willingness to be measured, critiqued, and challenged by those you love, trust, and even by those you don't even know. Thank them for their investment in you; it is worth it!
>
> —Tammy Webb, PhD(c), MSN, RN, NE-BC, Executive Vice President, Chief Nurse Executive

> Although much of academia is very social and collaborative, the writing process itself can feel very isolating. My advice is to (a) have a support person you can seek advice from, or maybe just vent to. My best friend is an academic in a discipline outside of mine, and our conversations (and sometimes vents/rants) about the various peer reviews we have each received have been a lifesaver because it helps me get the negative thoughts out of my system and see where I really need to focus for improvement. (b) Keep the big picture in mind: Your work is valuable, and reviewers want to help you improve your work. Even the most esteemed faculty receive difficult and challenging peer reviews, so hang in there! (c) Have gumption and get those edits back out the door. I tend to skim through the reviews immediately and then let the main takeaways marinate for a couple of days before addressing them. Even when it's just being in the exhausted

headspace of "What do I have to do to not have to look at this document again for a while?" get ready to jump in and tackle it.

—Katie Cooper, PhD, Associate Teaching Professor of Sociology

Five Stages of Grief After a Paper/Proposal Review

Critique of our scholarly written products can be challenging to receive. Before any writer can move forward and process the feedback, students should first try to set aside the emotions that may be surfacing. Dr. Tracie Harrison shares her advice for helping writers process the emotions and move forward to a more promising product:

The stages of grief by Kübler-Ross (1969) are as follows:

1. Denial (This isn't happening to me!)
2. Anger (Why is this happening to me?)
3. Bargaining (I promise I'll be a better person if ...)
4. Depression (I don't care anymore.)
5. Acceptance (I'm ready for whatever comes.)

We can apply these same stages to our emotional feedback when receiving a review for a manuscript, grant proposal, or any scholarly written product:

1. *Denial*: This is obviously a huge mistake. Maybe they got the manuscripts mixed up and the reviewer got another article or proposal. They couldn't be referring to my work.
2. *Anger*: The reviewer is an idiot! Obviously, they do not know what they are talking about. Why do I have to suffer with incompetent reviewers? I have read published articles that are much worse than mine. The reviewer did not understand me! If they would have read this more carefully, they would have liked it. Einstein was not understood at first either. I think he even failed math. If I ever find out who that reviewer is, I will snub them! Moreover, I think John Doe received a good review, and I know I am as smart as he is! Why didn't anyone teach me this in class?
3. *Bargaining*: Maybe they will fund it or publish it anyway. I will just call the editor or program officer.
4. *Depression*: I am a loser and will never get funded or published. Why did I bother? I am going home tonight to eat a gallon of chocolate-chip cookie dough ice cream. I will quit in the morning.
5. *Acceptance*: The reviewers were referring to my work, and they are not idiots. My work will not be published anyway. (The 12 calls to the editor or program officer

> did me little good. In fact, they mentioned something about a restraining order.) However, I am not a loser. I must admit, though, that this was not the best article or proposal. The reviewers were right about at least 7 of their 10 points. My work can always be improved. My work will be better if I address these points and submit it again. I am better for having had this experience.

Key points: There is an emotional/psychological component to getting your work critiqued. Allow yourself some reasonable denial, anger, bargaining, and depression but then move on. Your experiences being critiqued in class are frequently minor compared to the critiques you may receive from outside reviewers, but both help to prepare you. In the end, you will know you are growing in a scholarly manner when you hunt for those critiques!

—Tracie C. Harrison, PhD, RN, FAAN, FGSA, Professor of Nursing, and Alice An-Loh Sun Endowed Chair in Geriatric Nursing

Navigating Extreme Emotional Responses

Students can often get stuck at one of the stages described. Usually, students fall into the traps of anger or depression. Even faculty, who are regarded as experts by students can struggle with moving through their emotions from the reviews. This can hinder their writing process and may delay their publication acceptance. Delaying publication can be detrimental for faculty as many tenure and promotion criteria are based on number of publications per year. We discuss this point to provide you, the student or novice, with a look through the lens of even the most expert writers. If the experts have moments of emotional response to writing, then the process is certainly normal for all to feel at one point or another. Regardless of the level of expertise, all nursing writers (faculty, students, nurse leaders) may need to rely on peers or mentors to provide perspective when navigating the reviews. Meeting with others (e.g., mentors, faculty, etc.) who are emotionally safe and want to promote your growth and success is essential while moving through the revision process. We often encourage students to identify faculty who have a special interest in writing and mentoring students. The right combination can truly have a positive, encouraging effect for the writer.

> I was working on my first external grant application and recently received preliminary feedback from a set of internal reviewers. When I read their words, my heart sank. I spent so much time perfectly crafting these sentences and looking up the best references, but my effort did not matter. I was being judged on sentences and argument development ... and I felt so misunderstood. After sulking around for about 3 days (including lots of bath time, sad music time, and fluffy socks time), I finally got to revising my grant based on their feedback. But then, in almost an instant, I quickly panicked! There were so many changes to be made, and I was on such a short timeline. How was I ever going to fix everything? My 3-day sulk was totally pointless as I tried to work through the

> revisions. I was back to square one. Finally, I reached out to my mentor, and we reviewed the feedback together (especially the points that brought me so much anxiety). She quickly helped me to see what things were easily fixable and then identified the other needed changes based on level of difficulty. With her help I was able to work through the revisions from easiest to hardest, and this gave me the confidence to finish. I'm so grateful for my mentor helping me to see the true molehills and the true mountains. Without her I would've been paralyzed in fear and possibly not met my deadline.
>
> —Pearman D. Parker, PhD, MPH, RN, PMH-BC, Assistant Professor

Receiving Grant Reviews

Graduate nursing students and faculty often apply for internal funding (available to those at their college or university) or external funding (outside organizations, federal agencies, etc.). The grant review process generally includes a review prior to awarding funding. The reviews can be productive (offer helpful feedback for changes required prior to funding) or provide insight to the writer for why the application was not chosen for funding. Due to the nature of competitive grant applications, receiving the reviews can be one of the most challenging aspects of grant writing.

One of my friends and colleagues, Dr. Tara Johnson, told me the following over lunch once at a local café:

> I was sooooo upset [with my first grant application], and I thought that my career in academia was over, and it hadn't really even started yet! I called my husband, crying and said, "That one reviewer was so mean, and he didn't even read my application!" But then, my (professional musician) husband reminded me that he took 27 auditions before he won his first job. Of course, I was still angry, because it wasn't the same thing, and he didn't understand my situation!
>
> After I dusted myself off and read the feedback with a more level head, I fixed everything that that reviewer critiqued, [resubmitted the grant for another mechanism], and got it! In retrospect, I realized that the "mean" reviewer did me a huge favor by providing so much detail regarding what needed to be fixed, and I am glad that I paid attention to what he said. I still make fun of myself over that one!
>
> —Tara Johnson, MD, Assistant Professor, College of Medicine

References

Kübler-Ross, E. (1969). *On death & dying: What the dying have to teach doctors, nurses, clergy & their own families*. Scribner. Index

Index

Printed by Libri Plureos GmbH in Hamburg,
Germany